The Psychology of PCOS is a thorough examination of the symptoms of PCOS and their effects on the lives of those who live with the disorder. Dr. Williams clearly explains psychological research and theories to assist therapists who have clients with PCOS and to guide researchers to gaps in our understanding of psychosocial aspects of the syndrome. Individuals with PCOS, especially those who do not know others with the diagnosis, will appreciate reading excerpts from Williams's extensive interviews and learning about her own experience.

—JOAN C. CHRISLER, PhD, PROFESSOR EMERITA OF PSYCHOLOGY, CONNECTICUT COLLEGE, NEW LONDON, CT, UNITED STATES, AND FOUNDING EDITOR, *WOMEN'S REPRODUCTIVE HEALTH*

This exceptional, thought-provoking, and beautifully written book humanizes the lived experiences of people with PCOS. It moves PCOS into new avenues of scholarship by centering how we flourish and thrive with PCOS and create our own pathways to self-compassion, growth, healing, and community despite the challenges and complexities of the syndrome. It is the first book of its kind to integrate individual, societal, and community-level systems with the goal of creating tangible solutions for patients, health care providers, researchers, and PCOS allies to improve the lives of people with PCOS. I wholeheartedly recommend this book and believe that it will unite us in immeasurable ways.

—KENDALL SOUCIE, PhD, ASSISTANT PROFESSOR, UNIVERSITY OF WINDSOR, WINDSOR, ONTARIO, CANADA

This conversational and easy-to-read book fills a significant void in understanding the psychological impact of PCOS. Dr. Williams comprehensively discusses the scientific and social aspects of mental health associated with PCOS.

—ANUJA DOKRAS, MD, PhD, DIRECTOR, PENN POLYCYSTIC OVARY SYNDROME CENTER, PENN MEDICINE, PHILADELPHIA, PA, UNITED STATES

Dr. Williams uses an intersectionality lens to examine the psychosocial experience of living with PCOS and unequivocally illustrates how societal expectations and misconceptions about gender and weight have adverse effects for people with PCOS. This brave book includes surprising anecdotes about the lived experience of people with PCOS that both educate and elicit empathy. It should be read by students of psychology, health care providers, researchers, and anyone interested in PCOS or gender-related stigma. Dr. Williams's call to action will inspire researchers in psychology and other fields to explore important taboo research questions.

—**KIRSTEN OINONEN, PhD,** REGISTERED PSYCHOLOGIST AND PROFESSOR, LAKEHEAD UNIVERSITY, THUNDER BAY, ONTARIO, CANADA

The Psychology of PCOS: Building the Science and Breaking the Silence is an intriguing qualitative study that aims to increase awareness, intersectionality, and action in scientific research of PCOS. Rather than focusing on infertility and weight loss, as much PCOS literature does, this book focuses on stigma, shame, the inadequacy of research on PCOS, and, most notably, the often-overlooked subset of gender diverse PCOS patients. As the author states, it is a "manifesto" and a call to action for increased scientific study of a large and mostly misunderstood patient population that deals with substantial stigma in addition to myriad lifelong medical and psychological issues. Given the devastating effects PCOS has on the lives of both patients and the broader community, this book passionately and positively asserts a demand for advocacy and education and paves the way for an intensified psychological study of the syndrome.

—**GRETCHEN KUBACKY, PsyD,** FOUNDER OF PCOSWELLNESS.COM, MEMBER OF THE PCOS CHALLENGE HEALTH ADVISORY BOARD, AND AUTHOR OF *THE PCOS MOOD CURE: YOUR GUIDE TO ENDING THE EMOTIONAL ROLLER COASTER* the

psychology

of

PCOS

Psychology of Women Book Series

STACEY L. WILLIAMS, PH.D.

the psychology of PCOS

Building the Science *and*
Breaking the Silence

 AMERICAN PSYCHOLOGICAL ASSOCIATION

Published by
American Psychological Association
750 First Street, NE
Washington, DC 20002
https://www.apa.org

Order Department
https://www.apa.org/pubs/books
order@apa.org

In the U.K., Europe, Africa, and the Middle East, copies may be ordered from Eurospan
https://www.eurospanbookstore.com/apa
info@eurospangroup.com

Typeset in Charter and Interstate by Circle Graphics, Inc., Reisterstown, MD

Printer: Gasch Printing, Odenton, MD
Cover Designer: Mark Karis

Library of Congress Cataloging-in-Publication Data

Names: Williams, Stacey L., author.
Title: The psychology of PCOS : building the science and breaking the silence / by Stacey L. Williams.
Description: Washington, DC : American Psychological Association, [2023] | Series: Psychology of women | Includes bibliographical references and index.
Identifiers: LCCN 2022036053 (print) | LCCN 2022036054 (ebook) | ISBN 9781433837760 (paperback) | ISBN 9781433837753 (ebook)
Subjects: LCSH: Polycystic ovary syndrome--Psychological aspects.
Classification: LCC RG480.S7 W55 2023 (print) | LCC RG480.S7 (ebook) | DDC 618.1/1--dc23/eng/20220802
LC record available at https://lccn.loc.gov/2022036053
LC ebook record available at https://lccn.loc.gov/2022036054

https://doi.org/10.1037/0000337-000

Printed in the United States of America

10 9 8 7 6 5 4 3 2 1

I am writing this book for you, dear reader. I have been thinking about you for quite some time. You—the mental health professional whose clients are describing their polycystic ovary syndrome (PCOS) experiences and want to learn more. You—the social or clinical scientist whose literature searches have landed you at the doorstep of this common yet understudied condition. You—the person with PCOS perhaps, who, like me, may struggle with a set of symptoms that make you feel different. *You—the one whose child, or grandchild, or partner is dealing with PCOS and who wants to get a glimpse into the world they inhabit.*

I also wrote this book for me. *As a woman who was diagnosed with PCOS as a teenager in the 1980s and who has suffered mostly in silence since then, I have wanted this book, to help me better understand PCOS and to know I am not alone in my experiences. Now, as a social psychologist who studies marginalized identities and stigmatizing conditions, I offer this book to make visible a group of people invisible in society, by replacing silence with science.*

Contents

Series Foreword

When the Psychology of Women Division was approved in 1973 by the American Psychological Association (APA) Council of Representatives, it was a fundamental recognition that a neglected area of psychology needed a voice. Now approaching its 50th anniversary, APA Division 35, the Society for the Psychology of Women, remains committed to supporting and promoting feminist psychology.

One way in which Division 35 has contributed to feminist psychology is through the Psychology of Women Book Series published by APA. The goals of the series, according to the division handbook, include advancing and disseminating feminist scholarship in any arena (teaching, research, practice) in support of the division's commitment to social justice.

To date, there have been 17 books in this series, from the inaugural volume in 1995, *Bringing Cultural Diversity to Feminist Psychology: Theory, Research, and Practice* (edited by Hope Landrine), to the most recent in 2020, *Older Women Who Work: Resilience, Choice, and Change* (edited by Ellen Cole and Lisa Hollis-Sawyer).

The newest contribution to the series, *The Psychology of PCOS: Building the Science and Breaking the Silence*, by Stacey L. Williams, confronts a topic that has been largely ignored by psychologists and others interested in the psychology and sociology of women and those with uteruses. As Dr. Williams demonstrates, PCOS (polycystic ovary syndrome) has many impacts on the body that have implications for our fundamental ideas about gender and femininity. Dr. Williams outlines what we know about PCOS, with a particular emphasis on the psychological effects associated with this syndrome. She has interviewed many individuals with PCOS and uses these conversations to vividly show how the symptoms are experienced across different gender identities, races, and ethnicities. The author's approach is both critical of current approaches and hopeful for positive changes in treating persons with PCOS.

For more information on the Psychology of Women Book Series and other division publications, visit the APA Division 35 website (https://www.apadivisions.org/division-35/publications).

—*Irene H. Frieze and Margaret L. Signorella*
Series Editors

Preface

A Note to the Reader

To be writers, we must understand that we cannot write on the surface of things, but must dive deep into unknown waters in search of our own truth. If we deny fear or try to circumvent it, our writing will lack feeling and imagination, and we will fail to touch the universality of experience to reach our readers.
–Peggy Tabor Millin (2009, p. 191), *Women, Writing, and Soul-Making*

Admittedly, there is some irony that comes along with me breaking the silence of polycystic ovary syndrome (PCOS). Although I have long tried to use my voice in the service of elevating the experiences and needs of stigmatized groups, I actually have contributed to the silence surrounding PCOS that I describe in this book. You see, I *have* PCOS. I was diagnosed with PCOS at age 14 but chose not to talk about it until now at age 45. The math on that is pretty straightforward . . . 31 years *of silence* about my PCOS. My silence did not stem from the mere fact that I was diagnosed with a health condition. For me, the silence stemmed from the shame attached to the particular symptoms of this health condition. Growing up and coming of age with PCOS, I felt different from the person I longed to be—the person that the culture told me to be. The symptoms of PCOS—obesity, lack of menstruation, and excess body hair—caused me deep shame, wreaking havoc on my sense of self-confidence and social life. These same symptoms that gave my body more traditionally masculine than feminine qualities made me question the very essence of me—my gender.

I thought about writing a book on this subject for quite some time but never did because of *additional* shame I might feel once people found out about my PCOS. I wasn't ready to unleash years of suffering onto the pages, exposing my decades of shame and hiding. Now, I realize that writing this book is less about my readiness as a writer and more about what you, the reader, need to know. Having a larger purpose beyond myself has allowed me to set aside my fears to write this book. It was the spring of 2019 when I knew it was my calling to write this volume, and I had to break my own silence, when I developed what Cheryl Strayed (2012) in *Tiny Beautiful Things: Advice on Love and Life From Dear Sugar* called a "second heartbeat"—when one has a book inside of them, waiting to be written. The second heartbeat doesn't stop beating until the book is written.

What happened in 2019 to cause this shift? I was sitting in a conference room meeting with my psychology research students for our bimonthly meeting. It was the last meeting of the academic year, and for the first time in my life, I disclosed my PCOS to my students. I felt nervous, yet compelled to share. What ensued was something I could not have anticipated. Following my disclosure, one of my students—a trans man—disclosed his own PCOS. This surprised me because PCOS often is associated with women, and I had not heard about PCOS in trans individuals. He shared his personal experience of being a teenage female and having an impossible decision to make about whether he should take medication that would treat PCOS and therefore help his female physical body to heal or forgo the medication in favor of his gender identity to help his mental health. Then a second student joined the discussion, disclosing her PCOS and the challenges she and her husband had gone through trying to get pregnant—she did have a child, a result of in vitro fertilization. Finally, a third student shared that she had PCOS as well. Of the seven of us in the room that day, four had PCOS.

How is it that more than half of us had PCOS and yet we did not know this about each other until the very last day of our working together? Why did we not talk about PCOS—our experiences, our challenges? As a stigma researcher, I immediately assumed the answer to that question was stigma but had only anecdotal data to support the claim. As I began to consider the possibility of PCOS stigma, I reflected on my own PCOS experience and the fact that I hardly ever disclosed my PCOS to anyone. In fact, I actively kept it a secret because of the symptoms that challenged my own views of myself as a woman. Because I strongly identify as a woman, I worried that somehow PCOS meant that I was not one. I feared that if other people knew of my PCOS, they would assume I was not a cisgender woman (where my self-identified gender as a woman matches with my female sex assigned at birth). I held these fears despite knowing it is perfectly acceptable to have a gender identity that does not match one's sex assigned at birth or to identify beyond the boundaries of the pervasive gender binary that sees only two options for gender (man and woman). For me personally, transgender or nonbinary gender labels do not fit, even though there is *something* different about me relative to traditional ways female bodies express traits traditionally associated with womanhood that I can't quite put my finger on. At the very least, my body does not always correspond with the mental image I have of my psychological gender identity.

That spring, when I broke my own silence surrounding PCOS, I also embraced a new purpose as a social-health psychologist who studies stigma— to initiate a psychological science of PCOS, beginning with this book. Immediately upon starting this book project, I felt certain I was doing the work I am meant to do and that all my training and career and personal experiences were ultimately applicable to this purpose of growing a PCOS research workforce in psychological science. For this book, I collected other people's PCOS stories by conducting one-on-one interviews. The identities and confidentiality of the individuals I interviewed have been protected in the text. These individuals living with PCOS varied in age and whether they identified as cisgender women or gender diverse (e.g., transgender man, nonbinary) and other demographic characteristics (see Appendix A for a full description of the demographic characteristics and methodology for the study). By listening to the stories of others living with PCOS, I learned that others have had experiences similar to mine, such as this question about gender, as evidenced by the excerpt below from Tina, a cisgender woman in her late 20s with PCOS. However, the qualitative interview narratives also uncovered a diverse array of other psychosocial experiences, many of which I have not had and have not yet been discussed in prior research literature.

> It's something I've been thinking about, and it makes me feel like I might not be totally cisgender, but I'm also not comfortable at this point identifying as trans or nonbinary. But it's possible that I could. . . . I'm not a trans man. I don't identify as a man, but sometimes it doesn't quite feel . . . I guess nonbinary would be what I could potentially consider in the future . . . after some more therapy and self-examination. (*Tina, late 20s, cisgender woman*)

SOME NOTES ABOUT POSITIONALITY AND VOICE

I am a social-health psychologist. For 2 decades, I have studied stigma and its relation to health in individuals from multiple identity groups. When I realized that my work could speak to understudied experiences of individuals with PCOS, I found a new calling. So although I am a seasoned researcher, you might say I am an early career PCOS researcher. My approach to the book involved weaving together narratives from qualitative research interviews

I conducted (see Appendix A for my study methods) with what we know in the science on PCOS right now. However, I emphasize what psychological and other social scientists could bring to the study of PCOS. If readers are instead looking for books or articles on PCOS from medical experts on clinical research, I provide a list of suggested readings in Appendix B.

In addition to being a social-health psychologist, I am a White, educated, cisgender woman who has PCOS. Although I was assigned female at birth, and I identify my gender identity as woman, some of my physical characteristics related to PCOS fall outside of what is acceptable for physical expression of gender for women. At times, I have questioned my "fit" as a woman. I also identify as a lesbian and am married to a woman. I have found the label of lesbian most adequately fits for my sexual identity, although I previously was in a heterosexual marriage. Recognizing that all these qualities undoubtedly could affect this book, I intentionally tried to recruit individuals who represented multiple ethnicities, genders, and sexual identities. Still, as much as I sought inclusivity of language and content, my own experiences undoubtedly impacted my decision making in innumerable ways. I discuss this issue in more depth in the description of my approach to the qualitative interviews in Appendix A.

My approach to writing this book was mostly traditionally academic but with some personal storytelling about my own PCOS experience or perspective as a researcher. The integration of personal story into academic writing challenged me to get comfortable with voicing my personal experiences of PCOS. I fully admit that my own voice has not always been forthcoming in my life. Like others have so eloquently described before, our authentic voices may surface only when we are fully mindful and intentional. Voice may be similar to Parker Palmer's (1999) description of the soul, a wild animal that you would never find by entering the forest calling out for it; rather, you may see the wild animal, like the soul, out of the corner of your eye, after sitting quietly under a tree and waiting. I have represented my story and those of others as accurately as possible—to the extent that my own true voice and those of others showed up for truth-telling.

Obviously, there can be risk involved in sharing our voices. The silence surrounding PCOS does, at times, feel impenetrable. I hope that this book inspires you to explore this silence, and to reach beyond it, whether you are just learning about PCOS, wanting to study it, or struggling yourself with PCOS. As Joanna Macy (2007) described in *World as Lover, World as Self*, truth-telling is "like oxygen . . . when we help each other to tell the truth, and open to the feelings that go with it, we validate our common experience and forge bonds of solidarity" (p. 98). The voices emerging from the qualitative research in this book revealed multiple truths about PCOS.

Acknowledgments

This book would not have been possible without my village of people surrounding me and supporting me. To all of you, I offer my immense gratitude.

This book literally would not exist if it were not for Irene Frieze and Peggy Signorella—the book series editors for Division 35 of the American Psychological Association—who saw the potential in my book idea and encouraged me to submit a book proposal. Your expert suggestions on nearly complete drafts of chapters sharpened my focus and my writing.

Thanks also to APA Publishing and the helpful staff for a seamless publishing process. Chris Kelaher, who believed in and acquired this book. Kristen Knight, my editor, who made me feel seen as a writer by offering suggestions completely aligned with my vision for the book. Elizabeth Budd, copyeditor, who masterfully edited the text. Liz Brace, production editor, who turned manuscript into book. The anonymous reviewers of the book proposal and completed book, who gave generously of their time to offer expert feedback and suggested edits that improved the final manuscript.

My departmental colleagues and university, who provided me with the faculty job I love and that supports my academic writing. The sabbatical awarded to me in the fall of 2019 afforded me the time and distance away from regular duties to think up this book and propose it. Additionally, I thank the Research Development Committee for providing funding for the interviews presented in this book.

Friends who encouraged me during my writing process. Cindy Kelly and Betsy Kappes, who listened to my ideas while we section hiked the Appalachian Trail and others. Sharon Stringer, a fellow writer, who called me every other week to share successes and challenges in writing. Pam Murray, who always inspires me to find joy through work that speaks to my soul.

Friends and colleagues who generously offered feedback and suggested edits on drafts of chapters: Gloria Gammell (Chapters 1 to 3), Clare Mehta (Chapters 1 to 3), Emily Keener (Chapters 1 and 3), Bridgette Peteet (Chapter 5), and Sharon Stringer (Chapter 5). Your perspectives stemming from your own areas of expertise as scholars and writers were formative.

Sarah Job and Kelsey Braun, graduate assistants who edited transcripts and served in my peer coding process, and Kelsey Braun who additionally assisted with references.

My online book-writers group—Emily Keener, Clare Mehta, Bridgette Peteet, and Shannon Audley—who encouraged me to show up for untold numbers of "live writing" hours over Zoom to work separately yet together in community on our respective books. Our professional group has been one of the most rewarding elements of my career thus far. Your friendships mean even more.

My incredible wife, Beth Evelyn Barber, who was an immense source of support for my hundreds of hours of writing time and who offered her keen editorial eye by reading and editing numerous drafts. Thank you for taking on all of the "extras" at home, which gave me the spaciousness needed to bring my dream of writing this book into reality: poodle feedings, human feedings, pots of coffee—the list is endless.

Perhaps most profoundly and reverently, I thank the individuals living with polycystic ovary syndrome (PCOS) whom I interviewed, who gave of their time during a pandemic to talk with me about their PCOS experiences, some of which they had never shared with anyone else. I am indebted to each of you. I am additionally grateful for the responsibility entrusted to me, to represent your stories of struggle and growth in the context of this book. We, together, are breaking the silence of PCOS.

the

psychology

of

P C O S

INTRODUCTION

Why We Need a Psychological Science of PCOS and What This Book Does

The purpose of this book is to build a psychological science of polycystic ovary syndrome (PCOS). Why should psychology as a discipline care about PCOS? As you will read in this book, the reality is that individuals living with PCOS can have poor mental and physical health and experience a host of other negative psychosocial outcomes (negative self-beliefs, unfair treatment from others, close relationship difficulties, poor health care experiences). These are topics that psychologists care deeply about, and yet PCOS remains severely understudied in psychology. Moreover, because of this inattention, the lives of many cisgender women, nonbinary, and transgender individuals of various ages and racial/ethnic identities who are encountering this condition remain understudied and therefore invisible. Psychologists are working with these individuals in clinical and health care settings where PCOS may go unaddressed. Individuals living with PCOS are our research participants, students, colleagues, family members, and friends, and yet we do not fully understand how PCOS impacts their lives.

As the purpose of this book is to build a psychological science of PCOS, primary audiences for the book are scholars, researchers, and practitioners. Indeed, this book is part of the American Psychological Association (APA)

https://doi.org/10.1037/0000337-001

Division 35 (Society for the Psychology of Women) book series and likely will draw professionals who are division members and those who are social, health, and clinical psychologists. However, scholars from other disciplines (e.g., public health, nursing) and other areas of study (e.g., women's health, gender, and LGBTQ studies) would also see the relevance of this text for their own scholarship. A secondary and yet equally important audience for this book is individuals living with PCOS and their advocates. One of the realities that struck me when looking for books that could help me understand my own PCOS experience is that all the books focused on controlling or reversing symptoms of PCOS through exercise and changing eating habits. None of the books shared personal stories of how PCOS affected everyday life. I wanted to connect with others struggling with as well as flourishing in spite of PCOS. I wanted to make sense of my experience of PCOS and know that I was not the only one going through it. Despite being written with a more academic tone, I hope that individuals dealing daily with PCOS will find validation in the PCOS themes and stories shared within this book's pages.

WHAT THIS BOOK DOES

This book lays the groundwork for a psychological science of PCOS by breaking what I see as the silence surrounding PCOS in the discipline of psychology. It spotlights a wide range of psychosocial experiences that individuals diagnosed with PCOS may encounter, all of which are topics relevant to psychological research. I chose to focus on psychosocial experiences because the current published literature from a mostly biomedical perspective does not tell the complete story of PCOS. I based the chapters on the results of one-on-one phone interviews I conducted with 50 individuals who told me that at some point a physician had told them they had PCOS. In the book, I use research and theory from psychology and other social sciences to explain PCOS experiences described by my interviewees and integrate existing research and other information on PCOS (scientific papers, chapters, entire books, websites, and online articles) whenever possible. I use these multiple ways of knowing to ultimately highlight potential priority areas for future research; because this type of qualitative analysis does not focus on frequencies of reported experiences or representativeness, future quantitative and mixed methods studies are needed.

By no means is the range of topics covered in the book exhaustive. This text is not intended to be a comprehensive review of PCOS. You will note that the sample of individuals I interviewed is not representative but rather purposefully diverse to delve into the areas understudied within PCOS research. Also noteworthy, I conducted the interviews with individuals living with PCOS from February 2020 through May 2021. I recognize that the pandemic was salient in the United States and across the globe at the time of data collection and analysis (see Appendix A for additional discussion). Thus, I acknowledge that findings of interview data discussed within this book were both collected and reported in this context. Additionally, this context may have influenced whether individuals volunteered for this study—for instance, individuals with the most COVID-related stress may not have seen the study ad or had enough time to complete it. Context is an important element within qualitative research, emphasizing that there is not one universal truth. Consequently, much more than in quantitative research, results of qualitative research may change depending on the specific sample and context. As is further supported by the content of this book, I would expect PCOS experiences to vary across person and context.

When reporting the PCOS experiences of individuals I interviewed for this book, I describe them as *individuals living with PCOS*. Most published books and articles on PCOS describe those impacted by PCOS as *women*. I chose to use more inclusive language because, of the 50 individuals with PCOS whom I interviewed and discuss in this book, 50% indicated that their gender fit a label other than "woman." Of course, this number is not a direct representation of the population of those with PCOS but rather reflects my intentional inclusion of diverse voices with PCOS.

Because those with PCOS whom I interviewed were a diverse group of individuals who identified their gender as woman, transgender, transmasculine, genderfluid, or nonbinary, I differentiate cisgender women from gender-diverse individuals in the book. I chose the label of *gender diverse* as opposed to other common terms, such as gender nonconforming, because it is more expansive and does not imply a comparison with an assumed normative way of being (APA, 2015). Additionally, whereas *cisgender* individuals are those whose gender identity corresponds with their sex assigned at birth, the umbrella term of *transgender* (trans) refers to the various ways that gender identity might not map to sex assigned at birth. Although trans individuals can fit within a binary system of gender, such as when individuals assigned male at birth self-identify as women or individuals assigned female at birth self-identify as men, not all gender-diverse individuals fit this binary. An entire group of people identify their gender as outside of the binary system and may self-identify with labels such as nonbinary, genderfluid, or genderqueer. Thus, I believe the label *gender diverse* captures these varying identities. Admittedly, the gender-specific language used in this book may quickly become inaccurate or outdated. I ask in advance for forgiveness when my labels and descriptions fall short of the best identifications and experiences of those impacted by PCOS.

Throughout the text, I provide illustrative excerpts taken directly from interview transcripts. These quotes are verbatim, except where I have replaced conversational elements (e.g., "um," "like") that are awkward to read and detract from understanding the content with ellipses (". . ."). Alongside the excerpts, I also include pseudonyms instead of real names and use age ranges (e.g., late 20s) instead of specific ages. I made these choices to protect the identities and confidentiality of the individuals living with PCOS I interviewed. Although I also include self-reported gender identity with each excerpt, I do not include racial/ethnic identity to further protect confidentiality. Instead, racial/ethnic and other demographic representation are reported in aggregate in a table in Appendix A. Importantly, although I asked specific questions during the interviews, I coded responses across questions. Therefore, most of the themes are not attached to particular interview questions. Additionally, the themes that I drew from the interviews were present across racial/ethnic identity. I have noted exceptions in the text when cultural aspects of PCOS experience were discussed by interviewees. Finally, whenever available, I used pronouns self-identified by individuals I interviewed. In a limited number of instances when these were not specified, I used a neutral "they" pronoun for individuals who identified as gender diverse (e.g., transgender, nonbinary).

WHAT THIS BOOK COVERS

Because this book focuses on the psychosocial aspects of PCOS, I limit discussion of biological and more technical medical research, including it only to explain the condition itself. In the remaining seven chapters, I introduce PCOS and its symptoms and provide a critical analysis of the silence surrounding PCOS, including the silence of diverse experiences based on gender (Chapter 1), illustrate how PCOS symptoms are stigmatizing (Chapter 2), investigate diverse experiences based on gendered embodiment of PCOS (Chapter 3), describe social support and close relationships in the context of PCOS (Chapter 4), explore psychological risks of PCOS and evidence of psychological growth despite these risks (Chapter 5), examine the health risks of PCOS combined with the inadequate PCOS-related health care resources (Chapter 6), and call for interventions, advocacy, and psychological science to improve the lives of individuals living with PCOS (Chapter 7). I also include two appendixes at the end of the book to provide further details on my methodology, as well as to offer suggestions on further reading for those interested in additional review or more medically oriented information.

In sum, in the formation of this book, I relied heavily on an academic approach that integrated my own qualitative research study with what is known from published academic literature to provide a road map to begin building a psychological science of PCOS. However, the spirit of the book goes beyond the academic, verging on manifesto. As described by Breanne Fahs (2020) in *Burn It Down: Feminist Manifestos for the Revolution*, manifestos express rage and seek revolution; they are demanding, radical, impolite, and unapologetic. Manifestos express power and authority in a nontraditional sense, as a way for the voiceless to express their cry for change. As such, the spirit of this book is manifesto, a PCOS Manifesto that demands the silence be broken. I—no, *we*—demand to be heard.

1

BREAKING THE PSYCHOLOGICAL SILENCE

An Overview of PCOS

Releasing our truth is worth the risk because, when we give voice to our deeper truth, we effect change across seemingly impenetrable barriers.

—Peggy Tabor Millin (2009, p. 20), *Women, Writing, and Soul-Making*

This book is about PCOS—polycystic ovary syndrome. Specifically, this book addresses the psychological silence surrounding PCOS. What do I mean by "psychological silence"? Psychological science is silent because of a lack of research on PCOS. Additionally, many individuals diagnosed with PCOS are silent about the condition. Many physicians and mental health providers are silent due to gaps in understanding about PCOS. As a result of this silence, most people are unaware of PCOS, creating more silence. Thus, there is a psychological silence surrounding PCOS. This book breaks the silence surrounding PCOS and its psychosocial impacts. Together, the excerpts of PCOS stories collected in qualitative research and the existing PCOS and other published research underscore a need for a future psychological science focused on PCOS to promote deeper understanding and, ultimately, positive outcomes for individuals with the condition.

https://doi.org/10.1037/0000337-002

The Psychology of PCOS: Building the Science and Breaking the Silence, by S. L. Williams

WHAT DOES IT MEAN TO HAVE PCOS?

If you have PCOS, it means you were born with ovaries and that you experience at least two of the three main diagnostic criteria: menstrual irregularities (typically amenorrhea or oligomenorrhea, which means absent periods or ones that occur more than 35 days apart); hyperandrogenism (high levels of androgens such as testosterone or clinical presentation of acne, male-patterned and excess body/facial hair, or thinning scalp hair); or appearance of polycystic ovaries (Goodman et al., 2015a; Teede et al., 2018). The "cysts" on the ovaries are actually follicles that never fully develop to get released as eggs during the menstrual process and take on the visual of cysts in the shape of a string of pearls on an ultrasound. In the next section, I talk more about the varying clinical diagnostic criteria and their prevalence.

A common manifestation of hyperandrogenism or excess androgens in individuals with PCOS is hirsutism. What hirsutism really means is that individuals with PCOS have excess body hair located in places where males usually get body hair (e.g., face, abdomen, backside). The extent of the body hair is usually assessed by medical professionals along a visual scale called the Modified Ferriman-Gallwey score (Yildiz et al., 2010), as illustrated in Figure 1.1. As shown in the figure, hirsutism is assessed along a scale

FIGURE 1.1. Figure Depicting Assessment of Hirsutism

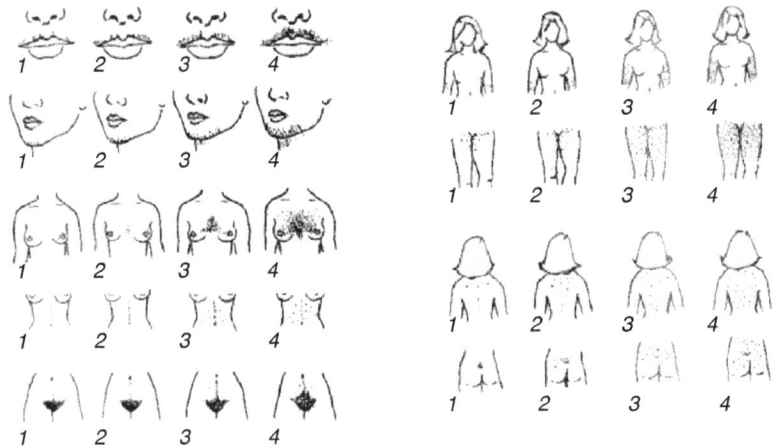

Note. From "Hirsutism: Implications, Etiology, and Management," by R. Hatch, R. L. Rosenfield, M. H. Kim, and D. Tredway, *American Journal of Obstetrics and Gynecology*, *140*(7), p. 816 (https://doi.org/10.1016/0002-9378(81)90746-8). Copyright 1981 by Elsevier. Reprinted with permission.

reflecting the extent of hair on nine different body parts ranging from 0 (*no visible terminal hair*) to 4 (*terminal hair equivalent to a typical male*). Scores are summed for a total that is evaluated against a cutoff score, such as 6 or 8, which may be indicative of significant hirsutism (although a cutoff of 3 may reflect hair beyond the "norm" for females and should be evaluated for hyperandrogenism; DeUgarte et al., 2006).

Although this scaling could be useful for understanding the extent of hair growth and presumably androgens present in those with PCOS, visual assessment might be difficult because individuals with excess body hair frequently remove it, and the use of a cutoff score may reflect more of the cultural valuing about female bodies and hair than actual biological abnormality (Azziz, 2018). Indeed, even the images used in assessments like that in Figure 1.1 are based on White feminine norms for bodies. As such, when interviewing individuals living with PCOS, I asked them to self-report excess hair rather than use this visual assessment. I also reaffirm the caution surrounding hirsutism that some might actually be normal variation. Still, more than 80%, or 41 of the 50 individuals I interviewed, self-reported excess hair due to PCOS.

Numerous other signs and symptoms have become associated with PCOS that might more accurately be considered metabolic (obesity, high cholesterol, high blood pressure, insulin resistance, or an impairment in the body's response to insulin requiring increased insulin production by the pancreas and which can lead to diabetes) and psychological (depression, anxiety, low self-esteem, negative body image, sexual dysfunction) correlates of PCOS (e.g., Teede et al., 2010), as some of these might instead be consequences of having the syndrome. The diversity of symptoms can create a unique challenge to PCOS because symptoms seem to vary from person to person. This variation was described by Jules, a nonbinary individual with PCOS in their late 20s who stated, "There's just as many shades of PCOS as there are people." This variation can also explain why PCOS is considered a syndrome, or a collection of symptoms, rather than a disease with specific and constant ones.

Take me, for example. I have irregular menstrual periods, having gone months at a time without a period. I am obese. I also have hirsutism and polycystic appearing ovaries according to an ultrasound test. In addition to the three main symptoms of PCOS that I mentioned earlier, I also have a compilation of seemingly unrelated symptoms that fall under the umbrella of PCOS that are related to hormonal and metabolic features of PCOS: insulin resistance, high blood pressure, sleep apnea, skin tags, and skin discoloration (formally called acanthosis nigricans) as a consequence of insulin resistance. Obesity, seen in large numbers of those with PCOS, is the central type, evidenced by a larger waist-to-hip ratio (Carmina & Lobo, 1999), which

I also have. Others with PCOS may report painful periods with excessive bleeding. Although not commonly discussed as connected to PCOS, some individuals with PCOS report a deepened voice, increased libido, increased clitoral size, and smaller breast size or underdevelopment (e.g., breasts that retain a more tubular shape found in earlier breast development), which may cause challenges with milk supply when breastfeeding.

I created Table 1.1 to illustrate the variety of symptoms and correlates of PCOS that were reported by the 50 individuals living with PCOS whom I interviewed. Everyone I interviewed reported menstrual difficulties, which is expected given it is part of the diagnostic criteria for PCOS. Although multiple cysts on ovaries (the "string of pearls" visual on an ultrasound that I described previously) are not a requirement for PCOS diagnosis, more than half (58%) of the individuals I interviewed reported having them. Indeed, despite the condition's name, some with PCOS do not have these cysts (i.e., follicles), whereas some without PCOS do have them (e.g., Polson et al., 1988). Further, there is evidence of hyperandrogenism in the individuals I interviewed, as shown by the frequencies of excess hair (82%) and acne (70%). Although symptoms vary among the diagnosed, a large percentage

TABLE 1.1. PCOS Symptoms Reported by Individuals Living With PCOS (*N* = 50)

Symptom	*n* (%)
Irregular menstrual cycle	50 (100%)
Obesity	43 (86%)
Excess hair	41 (82%)
Depression	40 (80%)
Anxiety	37 (74%)
Acne	35 (70%)
Pain	35 (70%)
Ovarian "cysts"	29 (58%)
Insulin resistance	28 (56%)
Skin tags	25 (50%)
Skin discoloration	19 (38%)
Infertility	16 (32%)
High blood pressure	15 (30%)
High cholesterol	15 (30%)
Hair loss	14 (28%)
Sleep problems/apnea	12 (24%)
Underdeveloped/tubular breasts	9 (18%)

Note. Polycystic ovary syndrome (PCOS) symptoms and correlates reported by 50 individuals with PCOS I interviewed. Other symptoms attributed to PCOS were less frequent: apple-shaped body or masculine body features (*n* = 3), fatigue (*n* = 3), migraines/headaches (*n* = 3), deep voice (*n* = 2), enlarged clitoris (*n* = 2), hidradenitis suppurativa (*n* = 2), excess sweating (*n* = 2), and increased libido (*n* = 2).

of individuals with PCOS demonstrate problems with ovulation and both hyperandrogenism and polycystic ovaries (e.g., Głuszak et al., 2012). As shown, many other PCOS-related symptoms (obesity, depression, anxiety, pain, insulin resistance, skin tags) were reported by the majority of individuals I interviewed. Other PCOS-related symptoms (skin discoloration, infertility, high blood pressure, high cholesterol, hair loss, sleep apnea, underdeveloped breasts) were less frequently reported.

Because obesity was self-reported by 43 of the 50 (86%) I interviewed, I also calculated body mass index (BMI) for the 47 individuals who self-reported height and weight to provide further detail of the weight-related experiences individuals with PCOS discussed during the interviews. I categorized BMI scores according to the National Institutes of Health (NIH) and World Health Organization (WHO) classification (see Table 1.2; Weir & Jan, 2021). I chose to include this information because BMI is still widely used in PCOS research and health care despite the possibility that other measures, such as waist circumference to assess centralized obesity, might be more predictive of cardiometabolic health outcomes (e.g., Ashwell et al., 2012). As well, in Chapter 7, I address approaches based on body positivity that are being explored as alternatives to strict weight-based measurement to reduce weight bias and stigma, also discussed throughout this book, to facilitate health and well-being.

Using BMI, 39 (83%) of the 47 individuals were categorized as overweight or obese. The average individual with PCOS I interviewed had a BMI of 36.77 ($SD = 10.02$) and would be considered obese—Class II, although BMI ranged from 16.80 to 63.90, and the severely obese category was the most common. Of note, some individuals (14%) I interviewed would be classified of "normal" weight, with one individual underweight. Indeed, these frequencies fit with prior research showing the large majority (e.g., 80%) of those with PCOS experience obesity, whereas a relatively small portion are considered

Table 1.2. Body Mass Index (BMI) in Individuals Living With PCOS ($N = 50$)

BMI	n (%)
Severe obesity (40+)	18 (36%)
Obesity–Class II (35.0–39.9)	10 (20%)
Obesity–Class I (30.0–34.9)	7 (14%)
Normative Weight (18.5–24.9)	7 (14%)
Overweight (25.0–29.9)	4 (8%)
Underweight (16.5–18.49)	1 (2%)

Note. Table includes weight categories listed by frequency and based on National Institutes of Health definitions. BMI was based on height and weight reported by individuals living with polycystic ovary syndrome whom I interviewed.

"lean PCOS," meaning they may have diagnostic criteria of PCOS but are of normal BMI (Toosy et al., 2018).

Because of the heterogeneity of the symptoms, some argue that the name PCOS is misleading—that it does not capture the level to which metabolic and endocrine issues are at play. Lobo (1995) advocated in the journal *Fertility and Sterility* that the syndrome be named *hyperandrogenic chronic anovulation* (HCA) to make central the endocrinopathy features of hyperandrogenism and anovulation. Individuals I interviewed shared similar sentiments. Cynthia, a cisgender woman with PCOS in her mid-30s, shared, "I just think that . . . there's not a lot of emphasis on the endocrine issue that happens with PCOS, but it is actually an endocrine disorder." Jackie, a cisgender woman in her early 20s, stated the following:

> The problem isn't really the polycystic ovary . . . the problem is . . . the deleterious effect of having high androgen and insulin resistance . . . the primary driver of . . . metabolic dysfunction from PCOS. (*Jackie, early 20s, cisgender woman*)

A consequence of the syndrome's name focusing on multiple cysts on ovaries is that it characterizes the entire syndrome by a single feature that may be unrelated to the condition (Lobo, 1995) and limits cultural understanding of PCOS. Individuals whom I interviewed, such as Cynthia, discussed that if people know anything about PCOS, it is that the problem is linked to ovaries and limited fertility (which also assumes a heterosexist/cisgender perspective); they know nothing about PCOS as an endocrine disorder.

> I think that [people] need to know that it's not a gynecological issue. And maybe one of the reasons that it's not, like, super "in your face" is that misconception that it is [a gynecological issue]. I mean, our society as a whole does not like to talk about vaginas. We don't like to talk about sex. We don't like to talk about what goes on in those regions. . . . Because of that, I think it's [PCOS] not very talked about very much. . . . I could see how women who have it feel . . . less of a woman because they can't have a child. And that also is part of society's pressure—women should be having babies. And . . . I'd like there to be a little bit of a big cultural shift . . . for that . . . by promoting it as an endocrine disorder, that it affects all these other things, and not focusing on it as your reproductive system is broken . . . would be a huge change and a positive one. (*Cynthia, mid-30s, cisgender woman*)

CURRENT LIMITED UNDERSTANDING OF PREVALENCE, CAUSE, AND COST OF PCOS

Regardless of the exact symptoms reported or the specific name of the syndrome, PCOS impacts many individuals across the United States and the globe. It is referred to as the most common endocrine disorder in women particularly of reproductive age and the leading cause of infertility among women (e.g., Azziz et al., 2004). But just how common is it? The NIH, in its report from the 2012 evidence-based methodology workshop, stated that about 5 million U.S. women of reproductive age (which would equate to approximately 7–8%) have PCOS (National Institutes of Health, n.d.). And a commonly reported statistic for PCOS is one in 10 women of childbearing age, although the original source of this information is unclear. However, individual studies report rates both lower (e.g., 3.4% Black women, 4.7% White women; Knochenhauer et al., 1998; 6.77% Greek sample; Diamanti-Kandarakis et al., 1999) and higher (e.g., 26% of a U.K. sample of mostly White women aged 18–25; Michelmore et al., 1999).

Importantly, prevalence rates vary due to different diagnostic criteria used. There are three potential criteria for diagnosing PCOS: NIH, Rotterdam, and Androgen Excess Society (AES). The NIH criteria, developed in 1990, combines menstrual disorder with clinical or biochemical hyperandrogenism, which means that it is enough for individuals to have a clinical presentation of hyperandrogenism such as male-patterned body hair without need for a biochemical workup. The Rotterdam criteria, developed in 2003, adds the symptom of polycystic ovaries (multiple cysts or follicles on the ovary that resemble a string of pearls), allowing a combination of any two of the following symptoms: clinical or biochemical hyperandrogenism, polycystic ovaries, and menstrual disorder (Carmina, 2004). Finally, the AES (Azziz et al., 2009) criteria are similar to Rotterdam but require hyperandrogenism be one of the two symptoms. As a result of this work on diagnostic criteria since 1990, recent advice published nationally (National Institutes of Health, n.d.) and internationally (International Guidelines for PCOS; Teede et al., 2018) suggests the Rotterdam criteria be used but with the addition that phenotypes, or the four types of PCOS based on the specific combination of symptoms identified, be specified. These types are A (all three criteria), B (hyperandrogenism and menstrual irregularities), C (hyperandrogenism and polycystic ovaries), and D (menstrual irregularities and polycystic ovaries).

Some work has compared rates of PCOS based on diagnostic criteria used, finding the Rotterdam and AES criteria, respectively, result in higher prevalence rates of PCOS than NIH. These findings support patterns from individual studies showing generally lower rates when NIH criteria was employed (e.g., Knochenhauer et al., 1998). Some of the higher rates reported (e.g., 20% or more) may have used only criteria of presence of polycystic ovaries on ultrasound, which may inflate the rate given polycystic ovaries can be present in those without PCOS (Michelmore et al., 1999). A subsequent meta-analysis of 24 published prevalence study reports has more firmly defined rates of 6%, 10%, and 10%, respectively, for the NIH, Rotterdam, and AES criteria (Bozdag et al., 2016). This meta-analytic finding appears to justify the approximately "one in 10 women of childbearing age" description commonly reported about PCOS.

Yet exact prevalence is less clear because presumably many cases of PCOS go undiagnosed. I was stunned when I read in Jane Kennedy's 2019 book, *PCOS: The New Science of Completely Reversing Symptoms While Restoring Hormone Balance, Mental Health, and Fertility for Good*, that 70% of cases go undiagnosed. This statistic stems from a 2010 paper that calculated PCOS diagnoses, contrasting three diagnostic criteria (NIH, Rotterdam, AES) in a sample of Australian White women aged 27 to 34, and found that nearly 70% of the individuals diagnosed with PCOS in their study did not have a prior diagnosis—indirectly indicating they were "undiagnosed cases" (March et al., 2010). As a result of the inconsistency, some choose to describe prevalence as at least 10% of women of childbearing years have PCOS and that this number likely is an underestimate given that many go undiagnosed.

Prevalence data also stem from study samples limited in size and representation. For example, one 2004 study using the NIH criteria for PCOS found an overall prevalence of 6% in 400 premenopausal women aged 18 to 45, with slightly higher prevalence in Black (8%) versus White (4.8%) women (Azziz et al., 2004). But the sample was drawn solely from the employees at the University of Alabama at Birmingham. Additionally, the study employed the NIH criteria, which may have underestimated diagnosable PCOS. Although other studies have drawn from more nationally available data, these data were based on visits to medical facilities and review of records for how many visits were PCOS related (i.e., not how many patients in general were diagnosed with PCOS). For example, Jason (2011) reviewed national medical and survey data and determined that five visits per 1,000 in those aged 10 to 60 years were PCOS related. Further, Sanchez (2018) found 306 visits per 10,000 in women aged 11 to 60 years were PCOS related (determined by a specific medical code). Others have written about the referral bias present in this type of PCOS research, where referred patients in research tend to have greater hirsutism, BMI, and androgen levels compared with individuals with PCOS not self-selected into treatment (Ezeh et al., 2013). Thus, more comprehensive and representative research on the prevalence of PCOS in the United States may still be needed to accurately report prevalence rates of this understudied and multifaceted condition. Although some authors have called for national surveys to include questions about PCOS so we can get better data (Sanchez, 2018), this has not happened. Thus far, the best statement on prevalence may be drawn from the document developed by international experts to provide guidelines on treating PCOS, which describes a range of 8% to 13% of the population as being impacted by PCOS and acknowledges that estimates depend on the definition used and specific population studied (Teede et al., 2018).

In addition to a limited understanding of prevalence, etiology or cause of PCOS is not entirely known. This lack of understanding was highlighted by individuals I interviewed, such as Eve, who described the lack of knowledge and research on PCOS.

> With the exception of breast cancer, I think conditions that affect women exclusively or mostly are wildly underfunded. Especially for something as common as PCOS, that's like pretty serious . . . it's not just having acne. It really dictates the way that people live their lives a lot of the time. It controls what they eat and how they move and how they have kids and their mental health and their physical health and it's not just the light cosmetic disease. And there's really no research funding to find out what causes it or how to treat it. (*Eve, late 20s, cisgender woman*)

Whereas we do know that PCOS essentially is due to a hormonal imbalance created by increased androgens, insulin, or both (Teede et al., 2010), we still do not know whether this hormone imbalance derives from an ovarian, pituitary, adrenal, or more general defect (Balani et al., 2013). Likely, the imbalance stems from a combination of factors involving both genetics and the environment. Because there is evidence that obesity may exacerbate PCOS and that losing even a small percentage of weight can have positive effects on the body (e.g., menstruation and insulin resistance), many, including health care providers, focus on weight loss in PCOS. Because PCOS is an imbalance of hormones that impact obesity, it may be unclear whether obesity is a cause or a consequence (and further, how those with PCOS are to lose weight to reduce their PCOS symptoms when weight is implicated in the syndrome itself). Yet, there also is evidence that those with PCOS are predisposed to insulin resistance that is independent of obesity (Goodman et al., 2015b). Indeed, there are individuals with lean PCOS or who are not overweight.

Limited Understanding of PCOS in Diverse Groups

Equally disconcerting as the overall silence and lack of understanding about PCOS is the assumption that PCOS is experienced only by women (cisgender and heterosexual may be the actual assumption). It is unclear whether prevalence estimates include individuals with PCOS who do not identify as women, such as those who are transgender men, nonbinary, or otherwise gender diverse. Indeed, rates of PCOS and its impact within specific populations such as trans and nonbinary individuals are incredibly understudied and therefore unknown. Some individuals I interviewed speculated that PCOS was more common among those assigned female at birth but whose gender identity is different than assigned sex. At this point, speculation is all we have to go on because no studies have examined prevalence in individuals of diverse gender identities. Additionally, some believe PCOS is an intersex condition, but, overall, little is known about this possibility. I delve deeper into these issues of gender in PCOS in Chapter 3, uncovering experiences of the gender diverse, which have until now been hidden, as illustrated by Emerson's quote:

> I think it would be super helpful for people to understand that . . . PCOS does not just affect . . . women . . . there's so much gendered language used when talking about PCOS. "It's a woman's disease." . . . I'm meeting so many trans men and gender nonconforming people who have PCOS. And I feel . . . they're getting erased from this experience. (*Emerson, mid-30s, nonbinary*)

Additionally, estimates of prevalence appear not to include older individuals outside of childbearing ages (presumably due to the focus on how PCOS may impact infertility in women of childbearing age), even though long-term risks of PCOS are chronic conditions (e.g., cardiovascular disease; see Chapter 6 for additional explanation of long-term risks) that only get more common with age. Indeed, individuals I interviewed believed that previous generations of their family members likely had PCOS but were never diagnosed. The complexity of PCOS as one moves out of reproductive age is not well understood, and symptom presentation may move from reproductive and psychological to more metabolic (Teede et al., 2011).

Also lesser known are prevalence rates based on racial/ethnic subgroups and geographic locations (Wolf et al., 2018). Some guidance acknowledges that health care providers should consider ethnic variation in the presentation of PCOS symptoms such as hirsutism and BMI. For example, more severe hirsutism might be found in Middle Eastern, Mediterranean, and Hispanic individuals (see Teede et al., 2018).

The Cost of PCOS

As you will discover in this book, the psychosocial costs of PCOS are great. Yet a complete understanding of these costs is needed. One strategy for considering PCOS costs has focused on health care expenditures annually in the United States, although the exact amount of health care dollars attributable to PCOS is difficult to estimate. First, there is the cost of health care expenses related directly to PCOS diagnosis (identifying and managing PCOS specifically). Second, there is the reality that PCOS has a much more extensive cost due to the increased risk for many other health conditions such as diabetes and heart disease. On the basis of these two sources of cost, a recent estimate puts the annual expenditures in the United States alone at $8 billion (Riestenberg et al., 2022). In their calculations, 46% of this cost was attributable to treating reproductive issues and 48% to treating metabolic and vascular issues. Although there seems to be a common perception that pregnancy is the main concern with PCOS, pregnancy-related issues accounted for only 5% of the total cost. Even less of the cost was attributable to initial diagnosis of the condition. Moreover, as the authors stated, the estimated cost likely is an underestimate of the actual cost burden of PCOS on our health care system and on individuals with PCOS, given that it did not account for other long-term risks of PCOS, such as mental health disorders and cancer, or other indirect costs, such as lost wages due to illness and quality of life impact. The estimate also was based on a conservative prevalence rate (based on the NIH criteria). To address some of this unacknowledged financial burden, a recent investigation calculated mental health-specific costs associated with PCOS and estimated that an additional $6 billion are spent annually in the United States due to the mental health disorders associated with PCOS (Bonner et al., 2022). To summarize, the cost of PCOS is enormous, and we still may know only a portion of the total cost, suggesting a need for greater understanding of the full psychosocial burden of PCOS in individuals' lives.

THE PSYCHOLOGICAL SILENCE SURROUNDING PCOS

Beyond the financial cost of PCOS and its correlates, the psychosocial burden of PCOS might best be understood in its context of psychological silence of PCOS. The final section of the chapter considers the outright silence surrounding PCOS within psychological science, which has led to a lack of complete understanding of the condition. Additionally, this chapter highlights the psychological silence invisibility felt by those living daily with a condition that is not fully understood.

The Deafening Silence of Psychological Science in PCOS Research

Although PCOS likely is an ancient disorder that has been around for millennia (Azziz et al., 2011), the syndrome was not identified and labeled until 1935 (as Stein–Leventhal syndrome, named after the two doctors who identified the condition; Stein & Leventhal, 1935). In the 86 years since then, a good amount of research has been conducted on PCOS but still has not permitted a full understanding of the syndrome. There still is no definitive cause or cure, and therefore treatments only serve to reduce symptoms. Although some researchers have begun investigating the lived experiences of those with the syndrome through qualitative work, most of the published work is clinical or biomedical research.

Moreover, psychological science is largely silent on the topic of PCOS. This disciplinary silence also (unexpectedly) includes feminist psychology and other subgroups related to diverse sexuality and gender—the very professionals who care the most about marginalized experiences. In my own career as a psychology professor since 2006, I have encountered exactly zero textbooks that have PCOS as a covered topic. To my knowledge, the only textbook that includes information on PCOS is the recent *Routledge International Handbook of Women's Sexual and Reproductive Health*, published in 2019, edited by Jane Ussher, Joan Chrisler, and Janette Perz. Part of the content of the chapter focused on menstrual-cycle-related disorders summarized the literature on PCOS as one of those disorders (Woods & Kenney, 2019). To their credit, the authors described PCOS from both a biomedical perspective and a psychosocial perspective based on reports in the literature on women's PCOS experiences. Unfortunately, their chapter reviewed relatively little psychological science on PCOS because relatively little research has been conducted.

In fact, while searching the literature in the fall of 2019 for papers published in leading feminist or LGBTQ-specific academic journals, my research revealed that zero articles on PCOS have been published in *Psychology of Women Quarterly*, *Sex Roles*, *LGBT Health*, *Transgender Health*, or *Psychology of Sexual Orientation and Gender Diversity*. When I conducted a combined search based on the keyword *PCOS* with *Psychology* in the publication name, only 11 published articles emerged, most of which were in health-related or clinical psychology journals. One article on PCOS was published in *Feminism & Psychology*. To ensure the thoroughness of my claim, I additionally examined journals published specifically by the American Psychological Association. I did find one article on PCOS published in *American Psychologist*. Upon downloading this article, I found it was actually a published comment about a previously published article on women's health issues pertinent to mental health professionals and noted that it had failed to include PCOS.

Thus, the relatively limited research on psychosocial implications of PCOS in the decades since 1935 (and for millennia if one considers PCOS an ancient disorder) both reflects and contributes to the silence surrounding PCOS. Given the omission of PCOS as a topic of study in psychological science, it should come as no surprise that individuals living with PCOS perceive invisibility or silence surrounding PCOS.

Individuals Living With PCOS Perceive Silence and Invisibility

In my interviews with individuals living with PCOS, I asked them to share what they thought most people knew about PCOS, tapping into their perceptions of the culture's understanding of the condition. The consensus was that the general public does not know much about PCOS unless people personally have it or know someone that does. When I further inquired about *why* people do not know much about PCOS, those I interviewed, such as Kim, described how "women's issues"—issues primarily affecting women or, more broadly, individuals assigned female at birth, such as gynecological issues—do not get attention. Eve described the challenges associated with the name of the condition, its invisibility, and the bias against women as explanation for the silence surrounding PCOS. Indeed, despite the many areas of life PCOS impacts, it remains known as a women's gynecological issue.

> I mean, if I had to guess, I would say . . . that it has to do with . . . misogyny. I think that it's probably a condition that has been relegated to . . . women's care, which of course we assume that women are people with vaginas and ovaries, but . . . it just has not been highly prioritized because it's typically been thought of as a woman's trouble. (*Kim, mid-30s, cisgender woman*)

> I think part of it is that it's a weird name and kind of an outdated name. Another part of it is that it's kind of an invisible condition. In terms of how it affects your health . . . it's a metabolic condition and/or affects reproduction, but . . . day to day . . . you're not calling out sick because you have PCOS. So [it's] kind of something that gets discussed between patient and provider or maybe with a partner or close friend, but it really doesn't come up in conversations with people . . . day to day. And, also, because it affects women. I think if there was a condition that affected one in ten men, we would all know about it in the way that like everybody knows about diabetes. (*Eve, late 20s, cisgender woman*)

Importantly, prior academic and popular press authors have previously acknowledged that conditions that primarily affect individuals assigned female at birth are understudied or not taken seriously. Dr. Joan Chrisler (e.g., 2011) has shown that reproductive processes are stigmatized and therefore avoided. Additionally, in *Everything Below the Waist*, Jennifer Block (2019) described this bias in health care against women and calls for physiological justice. Among the many examples in her book, she mentioned PCOS and its treatment as an example of how women's health issues are not understood and treated fully. Specifically, she described how the pill is the go-to treatment of PCOS even though PCOS is a metabolic disorder that results in an impact on the reproductive system. This trend of deprioritizing women's issues is not only relegated to reproductive health. In her book, *Invisible Women: Data Bias in a World Designed for Men*, Caroline Criado Perez (2019) brings together multiple examples and sources of data to make a case for a gender data gap, or absence of data on women, given the systemic bias toward men, and the consequences of this absence.

The silence associated with PCOS may be linked to the invisibility of the individuals with the condition. Even without me having to ask them, those with PCOS whom I interviewed regularly stated that they felt invisible or that PCOS was an invisible condition. In fact, Kim clarified that invisibility is the hardest aspect of having PCOS.

> I think one of the biggest challenges for me is not feeling understood by others, and not feeling seen . . . [if] more folks understood my symptoms, they might have more empathy. I feel like workplaces might have better accommodations. I mean, I'm able to use FMLA [Family Medical Leave Act], which is awesome to not lose a job, but also quite frustrating. . . . I think the system's already set up so that . . . "women's problems" are not given respect or consideration in a really male-dominated society. And so again . . . the condition is not very well known or understood . . . and I do believe that it often is dismissed as a women's trouble. (*Kim, mid-30s, cisgender woman*)

Reasons for the Silence and Invisibility Surrounding PCOS

Why is a condition with such visible physical features rendered invisible? Fisanick (2009) acknowledged the irony that the symptoms of PCOS are highly visible (e.g., obesity, male-patterned body hair and balding), and yet, because these symptoms go against societal expectations of women, individuals with PCOS are rendered invisible:

> The PCOS body has great potential to transgress the boundaries of normative femininity. In all of its hairy, balding fatness, the PCOS body represents a challenge to what is expected of the female body. The problem is that it lacks visibility. It is hidden within the matrix of cultural expectations, and attempts to make the PCOS body visible are regulated not only by society but by women with PCOS as well. (p. 109)

Indeed, society holds specific expectations about how women should look and act, and PCOS goes against these expectations. In their book *Woman's Embodied Self: Feminist Perspectives on Identity and Image*, Joan Chrisler and Ingrid Johnston-Robledo (2018) discussed current cultural beauty standards for women and how women learn of them, try to achieve them, and are affected by them. Current standards of beauty for women, particularly Western women, seem to reflect a White, heterosexual, middle- to upper-class, cisgender woman. This ideal woman should be thin with a small waist and hips and feminine in appearance, her body hairless (except for a thick head of hair), her skin blemish-free. Through the many sources of socialization (television, magazines, advertisements, peers, families, teachers) we come to know and internalize these gender-specific expectations. When it comes to PCOS, the psychological impact may stem less from having a medical condition and more from the specific symptoms of the condition going against attractiveness expectations, as described by Tina.

> I don't feel that I am any less . . . of a person or that there's something wrong with me because I have PCOS. I think that because so many of the symptoms present physically in a way that people can see—in a way that's considered unattractive for women, I think . . . that's when it starts affecting the way that you feel about yourself. But it's not necessarily because something is wrong with you. It's because society feels that there's something wrong with you. . . . It feels bad. . . . It makes me feel angry. . . . It's unjust. (*Tina, late 20s, cisgender woman*)

The invisibility experienced at the intersection of identities at the margins of already subordinate groups is at the heart of the PCOS experience for those born with female anatomy. Theoretical work and research on intersectionality (Crenshaw, 1989) may help to explain this invisibility. In particular, those born with female anatomy are perceived as subordinate to those born with male anatomy. Within these groups, however, those whose gender identity is different from their assigned sex or those whose gender identity does not fall along a strict gender binary, are marginalized. Individuals within a subordinate group who are further marginalized are rendered invisible because they are not the prototype of the subordinate group (Purdie-Vaughns & Eibach, 2008). Whereas some argue that the prototypical members of the subordinate group receive more stigma and discrimination from the dominant group, the marginalized-subordinate individuals encounter both stigma *and* a lack of recognition of their stigma due to their invisibility. As we will see in the chapters of this book, the symptoms of PCOS can render those with the condition marginalized and invisible. In the next chapter, I explore the stigmatizing nature of PCOS symptoms, which might help to explain some of the silence surrounding PCOS.

2 PCOS STIGMA

One Diagnosis but Multiple Stigmas

When we are experiencing shame, we are steeped in the fear of being ridiculed, diminished or seen as flawed. We are afraid that we've exposed or revealed a part of us that jeopardizes our connection and our worthiness of acceptance.
—Brené Brown (2007, p. 20), *I Thought It Was Just Me (but It Isn't)*

In Chapter 1, I introduced polycystic ovary syndrome (PCOS) and its varying symptoms. Additionally, I provided a critical analysis of the psychological silence surrounding PCOS. Perhaps helping to explain this invisibility, in this second chapter of the book, I argue that PCOS is stigmatizing largely because it comprises a variety of symptoms, each of which could be stigmatizing. In this way, PCOS may be a condition involving one diagnosis but multiple stigmas. Because stigma is a complex concept, I define stigma more generally before applying it to PCOS symptoms, using excerpts from the interviews with individuals living with PCOS to illustrate. I end the chapter with an acknowledgment that individuals with PCOS are likely experiencing multiple stigmatizing symptoms simultaneously.

https://doi.org/10.1037/0000337-003
The Psychology of PCOS: Building the Science and Breaking the Silence, by S. L. Williams

WHAT EXACTLY IS STIGMA?

To address the question of whether PCOS symptoms are stigmatizing, we must define stigma. In my 2 decades as a stigma scholar and professor, I have worked with many university students interested in studying stigma but who get overwhelmed trying to fully grasp the stigma concept. In their defense, stigma is complicated. The complexity lies in the multiple ways that stigma can be defined. Here, we focus on three. All at once, *stigma* can refer to a characteristic about a person (stigmatized characteristic), the way that others treat individuals holding that characteristic (enacted stigma), and the way that individuals view themselves for holding the characteristic (internalized stigma). The latter two represent stigma processes or how the stigmatized characteristic itself comes to impact the individuals holding the characteristic (Major, Dovidio, et al., 2018). In making a case that PCOS is stigmatizing, I will apply all three of these definitions to the symptoms of PCOS.

Stigmatized Characteristic

A characteristic of a person can be considered a stigma when it is deeply discrediting (Goffman, 1963) or devalued by others in a particular social context (Crocker et al., 1998). Although human differences are ubiquitous, society judges these differences and deems some as inferior. Erving Goffman (1963) acknowledged that this judgment from society is at the heart of stigma: "differentness itself of course derives from society, for ordinarily before a difference can matter much it must be conceptualized collectively by the society as a whole" (p. 123). Examples of currently stigmatized characteristics in society you are likely familiar with include physical disabilities, addictions, and minoritized racial/ethnic identities. Reflecting on these examples, these stigmatizing characteristics can further be classified as physical in nature as in the case of disabilities, reflective of weakened will or questionable morality as in the case of addictions (or other examples such as unemployment or homelessness), or group-based identity characteristics that get passed down over generations, such as ethnic identity or religion. For additional reference, Goffman first clarified these types of stigmatized characteristics and labeled them abominations of the body, blemishes of individual character, and tribal stigmas, respectively, in his groundbreaking text *Stigma: Notes on the Management of Spoiled Identity*. Thus, if PCOS were stigmatizing there likely would be evidence that PCOS symptoms are devalued by society and could be classified into one of the three types of stigmatized characteristics.

Enacted Stigma

Now that we have defined a stigmatized characteristic, next let us consider definitions between enacted and internalized stigma. *Enacted stigma* refers to the negative biases and unfair treatment from others that individuals with stigmatized characteristics experience; these can be explicit or subtle, intentional or unintentional, and can occur at interpersonal or structural levels (Major, Dovidio, et al., 2018). In other words, once characteristics are judged and devalued by society, they are associated with negative stereotypes or evaluations about the individuals holding the characteristics—beliefs and feelings that are learned and perpetuated merely by living in that society (Link et al., 1989). Consequently, individuals within society separate or distance themselves from those with the stigmatized characteristics, treating them unfairly, leading to status loss (Link & Phelan, 2001). Therein lies the enacted stigma.

Let me pause here and acknowledge that you may be familiar with terms other than enacted stigma to define similar experiences. That is OK. Different disciplines or scholars studying specific stigmatized characteristics (mental illness, sexual minority stress) may use different terms that have similar meanings. For example, other terms that similarly describe enacted stigma include discrimination, public stigma, social stigma, and distal minority stress. Please do not let that detract you from the main point here, which is that individuals can encounter stigmatization *from others*. Further, if PCOS were stigmatizing there likely would be evidence of enacted stigma attributable to PCOS symptoms.

Internalized Stigma

In addition to stigmatization from others, individuals may also experience *internalized stigma* or the intraindividual experience of adopting the negative cultural feelings and beliefs about the stigmatized characteristic (Major, Dovidio, et al., 2018). Because those with stigmatizing characteristics also grow up in society, they too become aware of the stereotypes and negative feelings about individuals with stigmatized characteristics. For them, however, these societal beliefs and feelings take on self-relevance because they actually hold the stigmatized characteristics (Link et al., 1989). In other words, they internalize them, taking on negative self-related perceptions and feelings of shame. Even when individuals with the stigmatized characteristics do not personally endorse the negative cultural beliefs and feelings, they can be affected by them in self-detrimental ways.

As with enacted stigma, different terms have been used to denote a similar internalization process: identity threat, self-stigma, proximal minority stress.

Again, that is OK. These are other ways of saying that individuals holding stigmatized characteristics can experience negative self-related consequences due to the personal relevance of society's negative beliefs and feelings. The main point here is that if PCOS were stigmatizing, there likely would be evidence of internalized stigma in relation to PCOS symptoms.

Additional Qualities

One additional point helpful to know about stigma is that qualities of the stigmatized characteristic can influence the stigmatization process—or how much enacted stigma and internalized stigma are experienced. Different qualities of the characteristic can elicit different emotions or behaviors from others (e.g., disgust, pity, distancing; Fiske et al., 2002; E. E. Jones et al., 1984). In addition to the three types of stigmatized characteristics already described (physical, weakened will, and group-based), the specific qualities of each of these types can vary. Although there are potentially many qualities of stigmatized characteristics we could differentiate (E. E. Jones et al., 1984), I describe two I see as particularly relevant for understanding PCOS, which are visibility and controllability.

The quality known as *visibility* differentiates how some characteristics are immediately known to others, whereas others are not immediately known and instead are considered concealable. Goffman (1963) first differentiated this quality as whether the stigmatized characteristic was discredited (those automatically known or visible to others) or discreditable (those that are more hidden or concealable but stigmatizing once revealed to others). Perhaps not surprisingly, the more concealable stigmas are linked to the ability to "pass" as "normal" or as not having the stigmatized characteristic. Individuals whose stigmatized characteristics can be concealed may go to extremes to keep them hidden and even experience what is referred to as "living on a leash" (Goffman, 1963) to maintain the illusion of not having the characteristic. Moreover, if a disguise or tools are used to hide the stigmatized characteristic, because of their association, they too can become stigmatized. For example, in some contexts, stigma related to old age might lead individuals to hide their bifocals that correct their declining eyesight. By contrast, individuals with stigmatizing physical scars or women with excess facial hair may hide their cosmetic makeup, cream, or equipment that disguises scars or removes hair, meanwhile remaining vigilant for signs these physical characteristics are returning so they can uphold the illusion.

Finally, the quality of stigmatized characteristics known as *controllability* refers to the origin of the characteristic and whether the individual holding it played a role in its development. In other words, if an individual's behavior contributed to the development of the devalued characteristic, there might be more stigma attached to it, whereas if the characteristic is perceived as uncontrollable, less stigma may be attached. In this regard, what really seems to matter is the perception of controllability by society, regardless of whether individuals had a hand in the stigma. For example, enacted stigma may be greater when others believe that an addiction is an individual's choice as opposed to viewing it as an illness outside of one's control. Similarly, individuals living with HIV experience more enacted stigma than individuals with a cancer diagnosis because HIV is assumed to be linked with risky or deviant sexual behavior or drug abuse, which are judged as controllable (Fife & Wright, 2000).

Now that you have sufficient grounding in what stigma is, let us explore the question of whether PCOS is stigmatizing. In the remainder of the chapter, I apply the definitions and qualities of stigma just reviewed to the symptoms of PCOS, illustrating how they are experienced by individuals living with PCOS using excerpts from the interviews I conducted. I chose to focus on the multiple symptoms of PCOS that are stigmatizing rather than the diagnosis itself, although the diagnosis of a chronic health condition itself could undergird stigma of PCOS. As outlined in Chapter 1, PCOS is a chronic condition and has no known cure. As opposed to the shorter time span of acute conditions, chronic conditions occur over one's lifetime and can influence an individual's anticipated life course, self, and identity (e.g., Wicks et al., 2019). Furthermore, when individuals experience characteristics that are biologically based, such as chronic illness, they experience shame that is about who they are as humans (Richards, 2019). In support of this possibility, individuals with PCOS have reported feeling *freakish* (Kitzinger & Willmott, 2002; S. Williams et al., 2015). This description presumably refers to the notion of being a "freak of nature," or according to the *Oxford English Dictionary*, an individual who is abnormally developed, one that may be exhibited in a show. Those with PCOS wish they were "normal" (Snyder, 2006) because they often feel abnormal, different, or unnatural (Pfister & Rømer, 2017; Thorpe et al., 2019). However, most of the references to feelings of abnormality in prior research actually stemmed from the symptoms of PCOS rather than the diagnosis. Indeed, individuals living with PCOS whom I interviewed clarified that any stigma they encountered was attributable to individual symptoms of PCOS (obesity, hirsutism, irregular menstruation, or infertility). Megan, for example, clarified that stigma experienced was not due to having PCOS per se but rather to the weight gain that results from having the condition: "I wouldn't say I've been treated differently because . . . I have PCOS . . . I think it's mainly . . . some of the symptoms . . . like . . . weight gain" (*Megan, early 20s, cisgender woman*). Similarly, Jo described stigma due to PCOS-related body hair but not explicitly to the PCOS diagnosis:

> I don't think anyone has ever treated me differently because they found out that I had PCOS, but . . . I was teased and bullied a lot as a kid because of being so hairy. And, when I had this job at an elementary school, . . . some other kids would make fun of me for having a mustache. (*Jo, late 20s, genderqueer/nonbinary*)

ARE THE SYMPTOMS OF PCOS STIGMATIZING?

PCOS is a syndrome comprising a combination of individual symptoms and correlates, each of which could be stigmatizing: obesity, lack of menstruation or ovulation, male-patterned body and facial hair, depression and anxiety, insulin resistance, hair loss (male-patterned baldness), skin problems (acne, discoloration, tags), and infertility. To test this argument, I applied stigma definitions and qualities to the experience of the three most commonly reported symptoms (obesity, hirsutism, and menstrual irregularity) among the individuals I interviewed (and that may be the most ubiquitous in PCOS). In this section, I describe previous research when available and use excerpts from individuals living with PCOS to illustrate this application.

Obesity and Weight-Based Stigma

Although not part of the PCOS diagnostic criteria, obesity is a prominent and common PCOS-related symptom that can be stigmatizing. Indeed, psychological research on weight stigma supports obesity as stigmatizing (Hunger et al., 2015) even if no research has directly addressed it in PCOS. Given the nature of body weight, obesity as a stigmatized characteristic would be classified as physical and highly visible (or, according to Goffman, 1963, as an abomination of the body and discredited). Although one could attempt losing weight to forgo the stigmatized status, the characteristic of obesity itself is not easily disguised, and so passing as normal weight is impossible.

Although obesity is visible to others, unlike other visible stigmatized characteristics (e.g., minoritized race/ethnicity), those with obesity are perceived by others as able to control their weight, thereby contributing to blame for obesity. Indeed, blame emerges from perceived controllability, perhaps rendering obesity a stigmatized characteristic reflective also of weakened will (or a blemish of character; Goffman, 1963). Jordan, for example, identified this blame as the hardest aspect of PCOS-related obesity:

> The hardest thing is—it feels like everyone thinks that all of the symptoms are your fault. Like you did something, whereas you find out as you do research, that PCOS is just something that happened to you and there's not really much you can do except for management. (*Jordan, late 20s, nonbinary/agender/ sometimes woman*)

Because others perceive weight as controllable and blame individuals for their own obesity, they consequently feel justified to treat them poorly. Such enacted stigma attached to obesity is evidenced in multiple ways, such as through widely known cultural stereotypes of individuals who are overweight or obese—that they are lazy, sloppy, unmotivated, unattractive, and less competent (for a review, see Puhl & Heuer, 2009). As well, individuals who are overweight or obese encounter stigma from others in the form of bullying, social exclusion, or unfair treatment in multiple domains (e.g., employment, education, interpersonal relations; see Major, Tomiyama, et al., 2018), which influence their social well-being (e.g., Rand et al., 2017). Not surprisingly, individuals with higher body weight anticipate stigma and rejection (Blodorn et al., 2016). Moreover, stigma may be both exhibited and justified by lack of antidiscrimination laws that protect other identity groups based on sex, gender, sexual orientation, ethnicity, and disability, for example, from discrimination in employment and other settings (Penner et al., 2018).

No published research has directly examined enacted and internalized stigma and shame experienced by individuals with PCOS due to weight. One qualitative study of individuals with PCOS did find examples of teasing and bullying due to weight or body hair as part of what the authors referred to as *sociocultural navigation* (Wright et al., 2020). This gap in the research is surprising because many individuals living with PCOS are overweight (Lim et al., 2012). Furthermore, weight stigma in general is widespread (Major, Tomiyama, et al., 2018).

Individuals living with PCOS whom I interviewed consistently reported enacted and internalized stigma due to weight. Narratives reflected an awareness of weight-related stereotypes, personal feelings of shame surrounding weight, and unfair treatment from others stemming from blame associated with being overweight. Kim, for instance, described how she felt judged by others for her weight that reflected societal stereotypes of overweight people. "I feel judged about choices, like things I eat or being perceived as lazy or particularly as a fat woman" (*Kim, mid-30s, cisgender woman*).

Similarly, Angelina spoke to awareness of stereotypes associated with being overweight based on her experiences of other people underestimating her due to her weight, with them questioning her intelligence or self-control. However, she further described feeling compelled to disclose PCOS as a legitimate reason for weight gain to avoid blame from others. This intentional disclosure may reflect a compensatory behavior similar to those under identity threat wanting to make a positive impression (Shelton et al., 2005).

> I tend to be pretty self-confident, but I think, though, that my weight sometimes holds me back or makes people underestimate me, because they think that because I'm heavy, I'm not intelligent or I lack self-control or that I am sloppy . . . people are . . . often surprised by the self-confidence that I have. That I'm not supposed to be that confident because I'm heavy. . . . They don't like my self-confidence. (*Angelina, late 30s, cisgender woman*)

> It's [PCOS] been something that I want to say [to others]. I like that I have a reason that I'm heavy and not just . . . letting people assume that I have poor self-control or that I just can't stop eating Big Macs, which is what a lot of people assume when someone is overweight. (*Angelina, late 30s, cisgender woman*)

Eve described her shame attached to weight that she explains is due to exposure to various sources of socialization into a fat-phobic culture:

> Weight is more of a struggle . . . there's more shame associated with that . . . fat phobia that's been ingrained in me and comes from a long line of people in my family . . . always . . . very conscious of their bodies and comments on other people's weight . . . and also hearing in the media and hearing it from friends in magazines and radio. . . . It's hard to escape and hard to change the way that you view yourself and your body. Like as much as we want to embrace yourself, embrace like body positivity and acceptance and love and like third-wave feminism, whatever, it's really hard to balance that with like wanting to be healthy and blocking out everybody's judgment. (*Eve, late 20s, cisgender woman*)

Maggie described the particular challenge of the culture's fat phobia and blame surrounding weight for those with PCOS, whose reality is a harder time controlling weight: "I think society's pretty fatphobic and also assumes that, like, if you're heavy, it's your fault. And that's not a nice space to navigate when you often feel like you have zero control over how your weight changes" (*Maggie, mid-20s, nonbinary*).

Individuals living with PCOS also experienced this enacted stigma due to weight in multiple social contexts (school, work, family), which parallels the general literature on weight stigma (e.g., Puhl & Latner, 2007). Megan's excerpt illustrates weight stigma in a college context, whereas Kim discussed the impact of this stigma in the context of employment. Others, such as Josie, mentioned unfair treatment in the context of family or social life with peers due to weight:

> I'm a geography major . . . I'm in the honor society and we always take a trip every semester . . . down to a swamp and we were canoeing. And the professor was concerned about my ability to canoe because . . . I'm overweight . . .

therefore . . . I might [not] have enough stamina . . . even though I've been kayaking all my life and I'm very good at canoeing and kayaking. So, in certain ways, people will treat me a little bit differently. But it's mainly because of the . . . weight. . . . I haven't had any . . . reactions to . . . the hair or . . . the different coloration of my skin . . . just . . . mainly the weight. (*Megan, early 20s, cisgender woman*)

Fat women are highly discriminated against by potential employers. . . . I wonder also if I've had job opportunities that haven't worked out because of my body size. I have a pretty clear memory of going to an interview and having one of the staff at the interview . . . couldn't stop staring at my body and . . . it just felt really uncomfortable and it felt very much about my body size. (*Kim, mid-30s, cisgender woman*)

Weight is . . . a taboo in my family, and adjusting to having PCOS has been hard for me because they always make comments about what I'm eating, even if it's considered healthy, or the way I look. . . . It also does kind of put a damper on my relationship with my parents because . . . they don't really understand and they kind of just blame me for the whole thing. . . . They don't . . . believe in it [PCOS], if that makes sense. . . . They . . . know that my doctor has diagnosed me with it, but they don't think it's real . . . they think it's just me being lazy or making excuses . . . I feel like people definitely comment on my weight, . . . even when I was in high school, they were mean to me about it. And they would constantly taunt me for it. (*Josie, early 20s, cisgender woman*)

As reflected in Jonny's and Alia's excerpts, enacted stigma was most salient after weight gain because it presented a noticeable change in the ways that others treated them after an episode of weight gain, also paralleling general weight stigma literature (e.g., Rand et al., 2017).

I definitely feel that being heavier, carrying . . . more weight, people definitely treat me differently. . . . I've been 140 and I've been 160 and 170 and 200 and 210 . . . I've had times to compare to . . . people definitely . . . treat me differently based on what my weight is. (*Jonny, early 30s, nonbinary/transmasc*)

I used to be slimmer . . . I was always what people would call "average weight." . . . But the moment I start gaining too much weight, . . . people . . . will not want to sit next to you on the bus. I've had people say very mean things to me in public—vulgar things . . . it's just really amazing how their attitude changed. If a man on the street wanted to talk to me, but I didn't want to talk to him, he would immediately go, "Oh, you're a fat so-and-so. . . . nobody loves you anyway." . . . It's . . . weird, because I know what it feels like to gain a lot of weight and how people treat you really badly because I became obese. But then I lost all that weight, too, and . . . people, now . . . treat me . . . differently, saying, "Oh, wow, you look so great." Some people that . . . weren't very nice to me, among extended family, were suddenly very nice. So I really have noticed how we, as a society . . . judge people based on something that honestly, I couldn't control. And I really see how unfair it is, and there's a part of me that's kind of blood boiling about that. (*Alia, early 30s, cisgender woman*)

Moreover, enacted weight stigma is woven into the very fabric of society, or, in other words, it occurs at structural or institutional levels, not solely interpersonally. For example, Dylan provided several examples of settings literally not being built with large people in mind and, as a result, individuals with large bodies needing to contort themselves to try to fit:

> I can't shop at the same store [that] my friends shop at . . . eat and wear what I want to eat and wear; navigating space . . . whether or not a tiny . . . café chair is going to support the weight of my body . . . when on an airplane . . . the contortions . . . to . . . get your butt . . . into the seat they want you to . . . there's a real maneuvering of my body to prevent discomfort and disgust from others. Yeah, I think a lot of it has to do with the way I navigate the world as a fat person. (*Dylan, late 20s, genderqueer*)

Although less frequently reported, the experience of weight stigma may be made more complex by the interplay with ethnic or cultural identities, especially when it comes from loved ones. One of the individuals with PCOS whom I interviewed spoke of this complexity related to being overweight as a multiracial individual, when weight-based stigma comes from one side of her family, but being overweight is more accepted by the other side of her family.

> My mother's side is my [one racial/ethnic identity] family and my mother's family is very anti-fatness . . . my entire life I was . . . made fun of and chastised for my weight fluctuating. And it made me feel very "othered" because, since I'm also [second racial/ethnic identity], I'm a lot curvier naturally than the rest of my family members. . . . I think that, naturally, I was predetermined to be that way, but also with having PCOS . . . I was . . . destined to be that way. . . . But it's . . . always been a point of contention . . . with my family members . . . fatness is a sign of being greedy, being gluttonous. So that's just always how I felt that I've been looked at by them. . . . Unfortunately, I haven't gotten to spend that much time with them [second racial/ethnic identity] . . . but overall . . . they seem . . . accepting of their bodies. . . . I've never felt uncomfortable about my body around them, . . . but I think also on both sides of my family, it seems . . . they've internalized a general American narrative of "we're supposed to feel bad about our bodies, especially if they're bigger than whatever the ideal is." (*Jordan, late 20s, nonbinary/agender/sometimes woman*)

In sum, the PCOS symptom of obesity fits with the definition and qualities of stigma. Excerpts from individuals living with PCOS whom I interviewed brought to light the multiple ways they experience enacted and internalized stigma. Clearly, future psychological research on stigma in those with PCOS is needed, particularly given psychology's long legacy of research in this area. Along this line, those with PCOS may be encountering a host of negative psychological and health outcomes that are implications of such identity threat and devaluation (Major, Dovidio, et al., 2018). A related research consideration might be the developmental timing of receiving such weight-based stigma. As one review of the literature noted, weight-based stigma experienced in childhood and adolescence may impede healthy development and increase risk for adverse medical outcomes already associated with obesity (Puhl & Latner, 2007). Many of those with PCOS reported being bullied or treated unfairly as children and adolescents, making this added vulnerability an important consideration for future research.

Stigma and Excess or Male-Patterned Body Hair

Next, I applied stigma definitions and qualities to another common symptom of PCOS—hirsutism. As described in Chapter 1, *hirsutism* is excess and male-patterned facial and body hair in females that is a clinical sign of excess androgens or hyperandrogenism. Considering body hair as a stigmatized characteristic, it would be classified as physical in nature and highly visible (or an *abomination of the body* and discredited according to Goffman's, 1963, definition). However, compared with stigma related to the visible PCOS symptom of obesity, hirsutism would not be reflective of weakened will because excess body hair is not typically perceived as under one's control. As a result, those with PCOS likely are not blamed for their hirsutism, as is the case with obesity. Indeed, there is some evidence in interviews with those with PCOS that body hair is not as distressing as weight struggles due to less blame from others for being hairy. One illustrative excerpt came from Eve:

> The facial hair and body hair, I'm better at accepting, because it's easier to just say "I don't care" and it's easier to hide and deal with . . . better than weight gain and difficulty losing weight as a symptom. And there's a little bit more sympathy there from other people. It's clearly not your fault, you know? . . . If you are overweight, there's kind of this nagging feeling that people think you're lazy or that you're eating too much or because you don't go to the gym, you're not as good or you're not taking care of your health. . . . Whereas if you have . . . a shadow of a mustache, people will be like, "oh, that's not cute" but they're not going to blame you for it. (*Eve, late 20s, cisgender woman*)

Although no published research has directly examined enacted or internalized stigma regarding hirsutism in PCOS, evidence suggests it impacts psychological outcomes (Khomami et al., 2015), which is covered in Chapter 5. The cultural mandate for female bodies (particularly Western European ones) to be hairless (Toerien & Wilkinson, 2003) contributes to the shame attached to excess hair (e.g., Keegan et al., 2003) and implies stigma. More than a mere beauty standard for women, hairlessness is a feature of the socially constructed notion of femininity or womanhood itself (Toerien & Wilkinson, 2003). Most everyone I interviewed described enacted or internalized stigma of hirsutism reflective of the cultural mandate. For example, Jo shared confusion attached to growing body hair in unexpected places for those born female, the challenges of being bullied as a teen, and the cultural mandate to get rid of body hair:

> Having . . . more male patterned facial and body hair has had a huge impact on my life. That was something I was bullied a lot for when I was younger, and it was really confusing to me because I thought I was a teenage girl and that I'd been taught . . . *this* is what happens to your body during puberty. And I was confused because they never said "oh, you're going to get so much more hair than everyone else, and it is going to be in all these different places, and you're going to get more and more every year, even after you're done with puberty." And that was really confusing and alarming, and I spent a lot of time trying to get rid of my body hair to the extent that nobody would be able to know I even had it. So, I feel . . . that's . . . a *cultural mandate* for people who are trying to pass as women . . . that you can't have even stubble in places that you're not supposed to have hair, which is pretty much everywhere except your head. And that's a really stressful project. It's a lot of time and a lot of paranoia to try and maintain that appearance, if that's not what your body is actually doing. And that was a big source of feeling invalidated as a woman for a long time. (*Jo, late 20s, genderqueer/nonbinary*)

Those living with PCOS felt shame attached to hirsutism, in part driven by images of the bearded lady in the circus and therefore desire to keep hair hidden from others. This particular reference is illustrated by the following excerpt from Sofia as well as limited prior published research on PCOS (Keegan et al., 2003; Kitzinger & Willmott, 2002; S. Williams et al., 2015):

> Probably more so keeping private as far as trying to get rid of the hair growth. That's not usually something that I talk [about] . . . different products and doing different things . . . getting rid of the chin hairs that appear . . . and the stigma of that. I've seen [with] circuses . . . the bearded lady . . . it really bothers me . . . the circus stuff . . . and the sideshows from years ago . . . and it having the bearded lady in it . . . she's overweight and she's got . . . hair growth, and you're thinking, OK, she's probably got PCOS. (*Sofia, mid-40s, cisgender woman*)

As with weight stigma, enacted stigma related to body hair appeared in narratives that described a range of social settings, such as school (particularly as children or teenagers) and family life. Indeed, several individuals, such as Juliet and Cody, discussed being bullied by school classmates for body hair. For Jack, facial and body hair was a huge source of shame when younger, and they reported being made fun of by their mother.

> Growing up, the hair was—was a very, very, very big insecurity for me. . . . I got bullied for it and called all sorts of names. Yeah, I got bullied very, very intensely in middle school. (*Juliet, early 20s, cisgender woman*)

And I got bullied a lot for hair growth when I was in school. . . . A lot of people noticed that and made me feel really bad about it. . . . I have hair on my face and my arms and my stomach and my back and my chest . . . it came in . . . when I was in the fifth grade. And kids are really cruel about it. . . . So when I was a kid, everybody bullied me and said that I was just a boy. (*Cody, mid-20s, nonbinary*)

When I was younger . . . the hair growth [was] a huge deal for me. As a teenager, I was extremely distressed by the fact that I had thicker, darker hair on my body. . . . I was teased all the time because I had darker hair on my arms. And if I didn't shave my legs, people would notice it on my legs. And it was a major source of distress for me when I was younger. And then in my mid-20s, around the time that I started dealing with more PCOS symptoms . . . I started to get the hair growth specifically on my chin. And I remember it very clearly because I didn't understand why it was there. I couldn't figure out why I was having hair growth there. And I was afraid to ask anyone because . . . my mind associated with . . . older women that grew hair in other places. So, I didn't understand why I was . . . 23 years old and having hair growth on my chin. But I remember it, because my mother, instead of saying . . . "hey . . . what's going on there?" just . . . made fun of me for having hair on my face. And it became a huge source of shame and embarrassment for me until I was older and I realized that it was just another PCOS symptom and that I could manage it . . . if I really wanted to. (*Jack, mid-30s, nonbinary*)

However, hirsutism may be less distressing or shameful when one removes hair and can pass as hairless. Although methods of hair removal such as electrolysis do not correct the symptom of male-patterned body hair, one can pay money for a service that will allow one to pass as hairless for a short amount of time. Because of the cultural mandate of hairlessness for femininity, hair removal is quite common among women in general (Toerien & Wilkinson, 2003, 2004; Toerien et al., 2005) and may protect individuals from stigma and distress. In a study of hirsutism among women diagnosed with PCOS, researchers found that although there were elevated levels of psychological distress in their PCOS sample, hirsutism was not a significant contributor (Keegan et al., 2003). Their qualitative follow-up helped to explain the finding by showing that women took measures to remove hair and to keep their hirsutism hidden from others. Because of stigma associated with male-patterned hair for women, individuals with PCOS concealed their hair growth to pass and maintain the cultural norm. The only exception to the stigma was related to women who held other characteristics in which hirsutism may be more acceptable, such as older age, being from another country, or being a lesbian.

Because with hair removal hirsutism shifts from being visible to conceal-able (or discredited to discreditable, according to Goffman, 1963), those with male-patterned body and facial hair may pass as hairless. However, this state of passing as hairless might require continued vigilance for evidence that hair is growing back and preoccupation with keeping up with their hair removal. To do so, they may go to great lengths to hide their hair and hair removal techniques, even avoiding certain social situations that may be more likely to show their body or involve bodily contact (sunbathing, sports; Barth et al., 1993). They may go to these lengths to avoid the interpersonal costs that would result from others' discovery of their hair (Toerien & Wilkinson, 2004). Furthermore, when individuals fear their concealed characteristic may be discovered, a host of cascading cognitive, affective, behavioral, and self-evaluative consequences are triggered (Pachankis, 2007).

Thus, individuals with hirsutism might not only remove their hair but also hide their need to remove hair. As such, the tools used to remove hair themselves become symbols of stigma. I will illustrate with a personal example. Because of my own hirsutism due to PCOS, I invested in a battery-operated shaver. I purchased it online, through Amazon, so I did not have to risk others seeing me purchase it in person. Whereas I thought I had successfully avoided shame by my discrete purchase, when the shipment arrived and I unwrapped the shaver, I saw inscribed on the tool, "Man Shaver." I immediately felt shame over needing this man-tool and hid the shaver in a drawer in my bathroom. I felt even more shame and embarrassment when my partner found it in the drawer and asked me about it. Up until that point I had hidden from her my need to shave parts of my body other than my legs. Apparently, it was obvious to her by my reaction that the shaver made me self-conscious; the next time I looked in the drawer, the shaver now read "WoMan Shaver." My partner's simple act of adding a "Wo" made my shame and embarrassment vanish. This story reflects the reality that to pass as hairless or keep up the illusion of not having male-patterned hair, one has to remove hair in private and with a continued vigilance so that others do not notice when it grows back. This need for privacy transfers to hair-removal tools.

Menstrual-Related Taboos and Stigma

A third and most ubiquitous PCOS symptom that can be applied to stigma is menstrual problems—amenorrhea or oligomenorrhea (absent or infrequent menstrual periods). All of the individuals with PCOS that I interviewed as part of this book reported irregular menstrual cycles. Although in some cases menstruation involved exceptionally heavy or long-lasting periods or continual bleeding for several months at a time, in more cases, periods were absent from their lives for months at a time. Like the previous two symptoms we discussed, menstrual irregularity as a stigmatized characteristic is physical in nature (or an *abomination of the body*, according to Goffman, 1963). Unlike the other two, this symptom is not inherently visible to others. In fact, concealing menstruation is not only possible but expected in our culture. Much has been previously written about how menstrual cycles are stigmatized, with population beliefs about them being that they are dirty or dangerous (Johnston-Robledo & Chrisler, 2013). A taboo exists about menstruation and discussing menstruation, which perpetuates silence and stigma surrounding menstrual cycles (e.g., Fahs, 2011; Johnston-Robledo & Chrisler, 2013; Kissling, 1996). This silence linked with internalized stigma attached to PCOS-related menstrual irregularity is evidenced by those I interviewed who felt shame and isolation from not talking about it.

> Before I was diagnosed with PCOS, . . . I really just felt like my body was broken. And I think I had a lot of shame around not understanding why I was having trouble with periods and what this pain was that other people in my life, who menstruate, . . . don't have. . . . So, what was going on for me? Why was I weird? And I think that shame made me feel isolated, because I couldn't talk about it or I didn't know I could talk about it. (*Kim, mid-30s, cisgender woman*)

Menstrual irregularity also is not seen as under an individual's control and therefore not worthy of blame. Rather, stigma of menstrual irregularity may stem from not living up to the expectation that all individuals with female anatomy should menstruate. Despite the negative attitudes and taboo about menstruating women, not menstruating may be perceived as worse than menstruating (Tavris, 1992). Menarche, or the first menstrual period, is a significant event in women's development. Within reports of the mixed negative and positive emotions women in college retrospectively reported about menarche, or their first menstrual experiences, were experiences of positive emotions of pride, excitement, happiness, and feeling normal (Chrisler & Zittel, 1998). Parallels exist in retrospective reports about menarche provided by women who had undergone hysterectomy. In her 2004 book devoted to understanding women's experiences with hysterectomy, Elson discovered that women remembered their first menstrual periods as the moment they became a woman and as both a sign of normality and their link to other women. Moreover, they reported a loss to their sense of femaleness that went beyond physical changes to anatomy or inability to have children after hysterectomy. Although they continued to view themselves as women after surgery, they performed gender in ways to appear more feminine and controlled information given to heterosexual partners to avoid rejection. Internalized stigma stemming from menstrual-related expectations was supported by individuals living with PCOS who reported feelings of shame as a result of absent periods, particularly at young ages.

> I . . . have never . . . had regular periods. And I've gone through bouts of . . . 2 or 3 years where I just don't have a period. And I think that I've felt shame about that . . . especially in my younger years when I saw all the girls around me getting their periods and . . . having it regularly. And it wasn't the case for me and just feeling like something was wrong with my body. (*Farah, mid-20s, nonbinary*)

The stigma associated with menstrual irregularity in PCOS also may stem from a possible consequence of it—infertility. Infertility, too, can be stigmatizing (Whiteford & Gonzalez, 1995). Although infertility may be concealed, it can become quite conspicuous with time if individuals remain childless. In addition, although infertility may not be seen as within an individual's control, it represents a violation of the cultural mandate for women to have children and become mothers (Becker & Nachtigall, 1994; Russo, 1976). Indeed, this violation can lead to enacted stigma toward those with infertility as well as those who choose to remain childless. The content of stereotypes or emotions attached to these two groups differ, however, and provide insight into the role of controllability. Whereas others may feel pity toward individuals with infertility (Fiske et al., 2002), they may have more negative emotions toward the voluntarily childless and perceive them as selfish for choosing not to have children (Callan, 1985).

When infertility strikes, the experience reflects significant loss and often a change in women's perceptions of themselves that corresponds with internalized stigma (Stanton et al., 2002). Feelings of inadequacy or inferiority can result when they perceive themselves as not living up to societal standards for women and, relatedly, as not living up to their own expectations for themselves as women. Infertility can permeate every aspect of life, resulting in infertility being referred to as a "master status" (such that its experience matters more than other aspects of life; Greil, 1991). In an in-depth qualitative study, women with infertility reported a multitude of psychosocial implications aligned with stigma: violation of societal expectation; feelings of inadequacy as a woman; lacking as a woman; feeling alienated or isolated from society; interpretation of others' behavior as belittling; desire to keep infertility a secret to protect self-image (Gonzalez, 2000).

Some individuals living with PCOS whom I interviewed experienced firsthand the consequences of infertility to their self-related beliefs due to violation of the cultural mandate for women to have children. For example, Angelina, a cisgender woman in her late 30s with PCOS, shared how infertility makes her feel about herself:

I can't have a baby like everyone else. . . . Sometimes . . . you just don't feel good about yourself. And the PCOS . . . the way it makes you look, the way it makes you feel, can make you feel just like, I don't want to say not a person, but . . . just not . . . a healthy being. (*Angelina, late 30s, cisgender woman*)

In sum, the experiences of individuals living with PCOS surrounding their symptoms (obesity, hirsutism, menstrual irregularities) fit with definitions and qualities of stigmatized characteristics discussed in prior theory and research. These findings presented in this chapter contribute new information to what is known in psychological science about PCOS. Beyond adding to the literature, it may be helpful for individuals to know that PCOS is stigmatizing. Although stigma-related encounters themselves are negative, explanations for unfair treatment that are external to the self can help the stigmatized to cope with these everyday realities of stigmatizing conditions (Major & O'Brien, 2005). Recognizing stigma can help to shift the blame for PCOS or its symptoms, such as obesity, away from the individuals experiencing it. Moreover, the invisibility of PCOS discussed in Chapter 1 may be explained by the stigmatizing nature of PCOS symptoms—symptoms that either violate cultural expectations or have associated taboos. For me, part of my healing journey in my own life has been acknowledging the role of stigma in PCOS. When I can remember that the ways others treat me due to my weight or the negative evaluations I make toward myself for my body hair are actually because of a complex socially constructed system of societal expectations (Toerien & Wilkinson, 2003), I am able to remove personal blame and shame when my body does not live up to them. Thus, viewing personal experiences of PCOS through a stigma lens may actually help to put a healthy distance between sense of self and PCOS-related symptoms.

ADDITIONAL CONSIDERATION: MULTIPLE STIGMAS

As we have discussed, PCOS is a single diagnosis comprising multiple symptoms experienced simultaneously. As such, an individual with PCOS may actually be experiencing multiple stigmas simultaneously. Individuals with multiple stigmatized characteristics at once can experience a greater impact of stigma. One possibility is that negative psychological outcomes increase as the number of stigmatized identities goes up, whereas another possibility is the impact may be based on the importance the individuals place on particular stigmas (Rodriguez-Seijas et al., 2019). A cumulative impact would imply an additive effect, with the amount of stigma increasing incrementally with each symptom an individual reports having. By contrast, taking into account the importance the individual places on the stigmas would require investigating the specific combination of symptoms and how individuals perceive them. The latter approach could account for social context and the centrality of the symptom in the individual's life.

Whether individuals perceive PCOS symptoms as stigmatizing likely depends on their other identity characteristics as well, such as their gender identity or racial/ethnic group. In these ways, PCOS stigma may align with the concept of *intersectionality*, which theorizes unique experiences at the intersection of specific identity characteristics rather than additive effects (Bowleg, 2008). An intersectionality framework also grounds PCOS stigma with a strong feminist foundation with roots in recognizing the underlying role of culture and structurally based oppression, rather than solely an experience within an individual (e.g., Collins, 2019; Crenshaw, 1989). An intersectionality framework could represent the complexity of lived experiences of individuals with PCOS-related stigma (S. L. Williams & Fredrick, 2015).

CONCLUSION

In this chapter, I provided evidence that PCOS is potentially stigmatizing because its individual symptoms, such as obesity, hirsutism, and menstrual irregularities, are stigmatizing. Moreover, PCOS is a condition of multiple stigmas converging within one syndrome, which also suggests that intersectionality undergirds PCOS stigma. In reality, PCOS stigma likely is experienced differently based on the unique set of symptoms each individual living with PCOS holds, along with their existing combination of identity characteristics, thereby grounding PCOS stigma in feminist intersectionality. Also noteworthy, this stigma attached to the symptoms of PCOS appears to be based in societal expectations, particularly for female bodies. Indeed, culture defines women by elements of their bodies (Chrisler & Johnston-Robledo, 2018). Therefore, in the next chapter, I explore a gendered embodiment of PCOS that considers the gendered nature of expectations and gender self-identification.

3 GENDERED EMBODIMENT OF PCOS

When the constructed status of gender is theorized as radically independent of sex, gender itself becomes a free-floating artifice, with the consequence that man and masculine might just as easily signify a female body as a male one, and woman and feminine a male body as easily as a female one.

—Judith Butler (1990, p. 9), *Gender Trouble*

Embodiment can be experienced positively or negatively, as empowering or disempowering.

—Joan Chrisler and Ingrid Johnston-Robledo (2018, p. 3),
Woman's Embodied Self: Feminist Perspectives on Identity and Image

Chapter 2 presented evidence that polycystic ovary syndrome (PCOS) symptoms, such as obesity, hirsutism, and menstrual irregularity, are stigmatizing because they violate societal expectations related to being thin, being hairless, and menstruating. In this third chapter of the book, I focus on the gendered nature of these societal expectations and how thinness, hairlessness, and menstrual function are expectations of womanhood. Because of this

https://doi.org/10.1037/0000337-004
The Psychology of PCOS: Building the Science and Breaking the Silence, by S. L. Williams

gendered nature, individuals with PCOS whose symptoms violate expectations may experience not only stigma but also a threat to their gender. Indeed, some of the individuals with PCOS whom I interviewed reported that PCOS symptoms posed a threat to their sense of womanhood and body image, contributing to distress. Yet not everyone with PCOS identified with womanhood. Individuals with diverse gender identities whom I interviewed reported that PCOS symptoms actually aligned with their identity and were an asset. These latter findings break new ground in PCOS research, which, to date, has focused solely on experiences of cisgender women and on symptoms that violate societal expectations for women. However, the idea that PCOS could be experienced differently depending on gender identity fits with classic work on stigma that specified characteristics only become stigmatizing when "incongruous with our stereotype of what a given type of individual should be" (Goffman, 1963, p. 3).

In the paragraphs that follow, I present evidence of a gendered embodiment of PCOS. Although not frequently used in psychological science, I chose the word *embodiment* because I believe it captures the close connections between PCOS symptoms and societal expectations for bodies, which are gendered. Embodiment or embodied cognition generally refers to the impact of the body on the mind, given that all of our experiences in the world are mediated by the body (Gibbs, 2006; Merleau-Ponty, 1962). When individuals' bodies conflict with the cultural representations of gender, their very identities may be threatened (Pounders & Mason, 2018). In their book *Woman's Embodied Self: Feminist Perspectives on Identity and Image*, Joan Chrisler and Ingrid Johnston-Robledo (2018) addressed negative embodiment specifically and how the female body influences women's sense of self because women tend to be defined by their bodies. Thus, a gendered embodiment may appropriately capture the interrelatedness of bodies, gender, and societal expectations when considering PCOS and its symptoms.

PCOS SYMPTOMS VIOLATE GENDER EXPECTATIONS FOR WOMEN

We begin with the undeniable fact that societal expectations for individuals based on gender are ubiquitous and can contribute to emotional suffering when they go unmet. In his classic work on stigma, Erving Goffman (1963) specified that one's psychological integrity was determined by whether or not individuals maintained such norms. Using expectations for U.S. men to illustrate the impact of gender violations, he described how any man who failed to live up to specific socially expected characteristics would likely view himself as incomplete or inferior. This particular example is relevant for our discussion of PCOS and gender. Applying this notion to U.S. women, it is commonly believed that their bodies should be thin, hairless, and fertile. Some expected differences exist among those of particular racial/ethnic backgrounds (e.g., more body hair in some), yet even those expected to be different get compared with Western European cultural standards. Furthermore, individuals assigned female at birth are assumed to have ovaries, to ovulate, and to menstruate. Further, the "motherhood mandate" dictates that females are to bear children and become mothers (Becker & Nachtigall, 1994; Russo, 1976). As illustrated by individuals living with PCOS in what follows, the implications for not living up to these expectations for female bodies are threatened womanhood, negative body image, and body dysphoria.

Threatened Womanhood

A common experience among individuals living with PCOS whom I interviewed was a feeling that, due to PCOS, they do not live up to the expectations of female bodies or womanhood—what I refer to here as "threatened womanhood." PCOS has been previously referred to as the "thief of womanhood" because it challenges the very notion of one's gender, leaving some feeling like "freaks" (Kitzinger & Willmott, 2002; S. L. Williams et al., 2015). At least 2 decades of research on PCOS from multiple countries have shown that PCOS symptoms of obesity, hirsutism, and infertility contradict expectations of womanhood (Kitzinger & Willmott, 2002; Naz et al., 2019; Washington, 2008; S. L. Williams et al., 2015), resulting in fear of violating ideals of femininity and normality (Samardzic et al., 2021). In my interviews, the threat to womanhood that PCOS poses was reported by individuals varying across self-identified gender identity. The following is an illustrative excerpt from Jo, who described PCOS as the opposite of the cultural expectations for women due to masculinizing symptoms:

> [PCOS] makes women the opposite of what we, in the United States, have constructed women to be, supposedly, because it causes like a lot of what we think of as more masculine features and for a lot of people it causes higher body weight and just everything that . . . we're told is the mainstream image of women, it . . . makes it harder to achieve that. (*Jo, late 20s, genderqueer/nonbinary*)

Tina further clarified that the *only* reason she feels bad about herself is because society tells her that PCOS symptoms run contrary to what is deemed attractive for women. These societal judgments create negative self-perceptions in those with PCOS who otherwise would not feel bad about themselves. This point is driven home by Jules, who described being told directly by others that their body violated gender expectations. Such encounters confirm the broad societal messages that contribute to internalization of expectations, resulting in shame and negative body image when PCOS bodies violate them.

> I don't feel that I am any lesser of a person or that there's something wrong with me because I have PCOS. I think that because so many of the symptoms present physically, in a way that people can see, in a way that's considered unattractive for women. I think that that's when it starts affecting the way that you feel about yourself. But it's not necessarily because something is wrong with you. It's because society feels that there's something wrong with you. . . . It makes me feel angry a lot of the time. It feels unjust. (*Tina, late 20s, cisgender woman*)

> I had such low self-confidence and feeling very unattractive because I'd basically been told my entire life that I didn't fit what was considered attractive nor what fit as woman. (*Jules, late 20s, nonbinary*)

Although not commonly reported, some felt their racial/ethnic identification made the experience of violating gender expectations due to PCOS more challenging because these expectations are based on White women. Jean, a woman of color, described how gender expectations were intertwined with racial identity, sharing how she already did not fit with larger cultural expectations for women and femininity due to her racial identity, further compounding the negative experience of PCOS:

> I also think that some of my feelings about my symptoms, and what it means for my gender identity, and what I'm allowed to do, and my gender expression also is connected to my racial identity . . . growing up in very White spaces and . . . navigating the fact that already, the ideals of femininity and being a girl and being a woman don't include me. And so then to also have . . . excess hair or . . . periods are weird and don't always come . . . made me feel like even a step further back from that. . . . When I was . . . in middle school . . . I really . . . struggled with this idea of . . . "am I enough of a girl?" . . . I was in dance class from the time I was 3 until I was about 10 and the last dance school that I went to was very exclusionary. And I always very much got the sense there that I wasn't a girl in the right way, in order to be considered . . . a real dancer. And so then with my period and with my body hair, . . . I remember in sixth and seventh grade . . . really rejecting a lot of femininity . . . because I was like—I don't think I'm allowed to be a girl. I don't think I'm allowed to be . . . a feminine girl completely. . . . I have to limit the amount that I do because that's all that I'm allowed to have because . . . the ideal of femininity is . . . some pretty blond White girl. (*Jean, late 20s, cisgender woman*)

In addition to these general reports of PCOS threatening womanhood and gender, individuals highlighted specific PCOS symptoms as being problematic for perceived womanhood. Hirsutism, or excess or male-patterned body and facial hair, in particular seemed to challenge expectations for the female body, leading to threatened womanhood. For example, Megan described the challenge of feeling masculine due to having sideburns and not wanting to look and feel like a man:

> I feel like PCOS really makes me feel much more masculine than I want to. I mean, I feel feminine, I identify with feminine traits, I identify as female, but I feel like people will see . . . these really masculine traits. . . . I have very prominent sideburns, which I'm getting removed by laser treatment because it just—it makes me feel like I look like a man. And I don't want to look like a man. I feel like PCOS mainly makes me look—or it makes me feel like I look very masculine. (*Megan, early 20s, cisgender woman*)

The salience of hirsutism in threatened womanhood is supported by previous published research on PCOS showing that excess hair contributed to women feeling less feminine and more freakish. Indeed, prior studies of women with PCOS have evidenced the challenge that hirsutism presents for perceived womanhood, thereby affirming the expectation that for women to be normal, they must have hairless bodies (e.g., Keegan et al., 2003; Kitzinger & Willmott, 2002; Pfister & Rømer, 2017).

Other PCOS symptoms that arose as contributing to threatened womanhood included infertility and body shape. As described in Chapter 2, menstruation and motherhood are associated with womanhood, when those with PCOS experience menstrual irregularities or infertility as a result of them, individuals may perceive deficiencies in themselves and their own womanhood. As illustrated by Angelina's excerpt, infertility goes against a woman's biology and purpose, leading her to feel less than a woman:

> It makes me frustrated and angry that my body won't do what it's supposed to do. That I can't. . . . I can't shop in the same stores as everyone else. I can't have a baby like everyone else. I can't get pregnant, which is . . . my entire function. Like that's your entire function. A uterus is to get pregnant . . . the infertility can make you feel like not as much of a woman because you can't do what women do. (*Angelina, late 30s, cisgender woman*)

Although increased weight or obesity is often discussed as problematic in those with PCOS, the threat to womanhood may also be tied to body shape. Women's attractiveness is negatively related to waist-to-hip ratio (WHR; measured by dividing waist circumference by hip circumference) in addition to lower weight (typically assessed by body mass index [BMI]; weight divided by height). Females with BMI and WHR that are low but within the normal range are deemed more attractive (for review, see Weeden & Sabini, 2005). Lower WHR indicates that women's hips are wider than their waists, giving them a pear or hourglass, rather than apple shape more typical of PCOS. Individuals with PCOS often are depicted as having an apple-shaped body, implying a more masculine presentation (smaller breasts and hips, larger stomach). This apple shape may be partially explained by increased testosterone associated with PCOS. Hormones play a role in body shape, with circulating estrogen associated with fat distribution in the hip area and circulating testosterone, fat distribution in the waist (e.g., de Ridder et al., 1990; Mondragón-Ceballos et al., 2015; van Anders & Hampson, 2005). Jonny described the feeling of not living up to gender expectations for females as alienation from womanhood due to the combined experiences of masculine body shape and hair:

> I didn't feel like I had the full woman experience . . . there was a lot that I couldn't relate to . . . the hair . . . kind of left me feeling alienated from, like the typical female experience. . . . It's definitely impacted my gender . . . which is also an interesting thing because . . . I fought it for so long, like having hair and . . . a male body type . . . I don't have super typical . . . feminine curves. . . . I carry a lot of weight in my torso. . . . And so . . . don't feel . . . classically feminine or attractive to people that like feminine people. . . . Up until before I really explored my gender identity, I felt incredibly not good enough, incredibly self-conscious. I felt like I said, very alienated from like being a woman, and—because—specifically because of the hair, because of the body hair. (*Jonny, early 30s, nonbinary/transmasc*)

Body Image and Dysphoria

Violating societal expectations for female bodies and womanhood likely underlies the negative body image and related distress encountered by individuals living with PCOS. Prior psychological research has found that those with PCOS are at particular risk for poor body image, or negative perceptions and feelings about one's body size, attractiveness, or body shape (Grogan, 2006). In fact, those with PCOS appear to have worse perceptions of their appearance and with specific body parts, compared with nonpatient community individuals and those experiencing infertility without PCOS (Himelein & Thatcher, 2006a). Thus, body image likely is intricately intertwined with PCOS symptoms that are gender violations. This notion also fits with classic work specifying that stigma varies by how "ugly" characteristics are in the eyes of society (E. E. Jones et al., 1984).

The interviews I conducted with individuals living with PCOS support this prior work showing negative body image. Many individuals reported dissatisfaction with their bodies. One illustrative excerpt came from Emerson, who described extreme dissatisfaction with body shape due to PCOS:

> I think this is something that I've been . . . dealing with . . . a lot lately, thinking about . . . my gender and how I feel about . . . my body, because I've never felt good about my body. I feel like I've always been at odds with my body. . . . But also . . . the shape of my body, . . . has always just been this huge . . . source of . . . insecurity. And, . . . even from . . . a very . . . young age, . . . my mom had . . . a family friend who . . . told me I had . . . shoulders like a linebacker. And that's . . . a really hard thing to hear when . . . you are a young girl who just wants to be feminine and pretty and small and . . . not being . . . any of those things. Because I did always . . . identify . . . with being feminine and . . . with . . . few exceptions, . . . I was obsessed with Barbies and Disney princesses and . . . everything I owned was pink and purple by choice . . . and just feeling like I have this body that . . . wanted me to grow facial hair and be shaped like a guy—or . . . what I felt . . . was shaped like a guy. (*Emerson, mid-30s, nonbinary*)

This body dissatisfaction stemming from individuals' bodies not living up to gender-related societal expectations verged on dysphoric experiences. Admittedly, I use the word *dysphoria* with some caution. You may be familiar with the term *gender dysphoria*, which references a clinical diagnosis. Specifically, the diagnosis requires clinically relevant distress or functional impairment attached to incongruence between natal sex and one's experienced gender for at least 6 months (American Psychiatric Association, 2013), although the newest *International and Statistical Classification of Diseases (ICD-11)* includes a shift from dysphoria to incongruence, redefining gender identity related mental disorders as sexual health conditions (World Health Organization, n.d.). To clarify, I am not suggesting that individuals living with PCOS are reaching a clinical definition of gender dysphoria. Rather, the experiences reported by individuals living with PCOS align with a more general term *dysphoria*, which refers to general feelings of discomfort.

However, I retained the word *dysphoria* rather than a broader term like *distress* because, in actuality, the reports of experiences of those with PCOS whom I interviewed were perhaps a mix of dysphoria and gender dysphoria. Whereas only one interviewee indicated having a diagnosis of gender dysphoria, many of the interviewees spoke of feelings that reflect dysphoria more generally. Further, because the discomfort or distress is related to violations in gender expectations, some experiences may verge on gender dysphoria even though no clinical diagnosis is present. To illustrate, I provide here a few examples that show the ways individuals described their dysphoria either directly or indirectly. For example, Jules directly referenced dysphoria related to PCOS:

> I think dysphoria is a very multifaceted and complicated thing that can manifest in many different ways for many different people at many different times. . . . And for some, not at all. . . . But . . . for me . . . dysphoria has really been present in my life, has really been intrinsically tied to the symptoms of PCOS. (*Jules, late 20s, nonbinary*)

Although Emerson did not state dysphoria explicitly, she described a recognition that her external body (due to body hair and masculine shape due to PCOS) was different from her internal gender:

> I just felt . . . it [PCOS] made me look like on the outside . . . the opposite of how I felt on the inside. And . . . that's just been this struggle that I've had . . . my whole life. And . . . then . . . I really let go [of] wanting to have a child and . . . I feel like PCOS has in some ways . . . locked me out of this experience that other quote–unquote, women have. Because . . . you don't get to look feminine, you don't get to look pretty and you don't even get to have a baby. And . . . that's really hard. And it really sucks. (*Emerson, mid-30s, nonbinary*)

Josie's experience verged on dysphoria because of the masculinizing features of PCOS that led to confusion and questioning of her gender identification. Her masculine traits and confusion related to gender were quite disturbing for her. As depicted in her second excerpt, she considered them taboo to talk about, even to her therapist:

> Yes, sometimes I wonder if it would be better for me to be a man rather than a woman. I think about it a lot, actually. I don't think I would ever transition or consider myself male. But it is something I think about. I have always had more masculine traits . . . even when I was younger, because I grew up around four older brothers. And this kind of just adds to the confusion of whether or not I'm actually a girl or not. I have higher testosterone than what would be considered normal for a woman. So that definitely contributes to me feeling more masculine and [is] kind of confusing [to] my gender identity. (*Josie, early 20s, cisgender woman*)

> It's very taboo and I am still trying to come to terms with the fact that these thoughts are completely normal. And I'm not the only person who thinks this way, and I'm kind of a little scared to talk to my therapist about it because it's something I've never talked about with anyone, because I'm afraid that people will judge me or say I'm confused or just crazy for the most part. I don't think my therapist would ever call me crazy, but I'm scared of her reaction and I'm scared of other people's reaction. (*Josie, early 20s, cisgender woman*)

Similarly, Tina self-identified as a cisgender woman, but described *feeling* "not quite" cisgender and yet not clearly identifying as transgender, illustrating the complex relation between PCOS and perceived gender:

I will say it makes me want to have a penis. I just so wish that I had a penis instead of a uterus and a vagina. It just feels like it would relieve so many issues. I am truly envious of people who have penises. . . . It's something I've been thinking about, and it makes me feel like I might not be totally cisgender, but I'm also not comfortable at this point identifying as trans or nonbinary. But it's possible that I could. I don't think I—I'm not a trans man. I don't identify as a man, but sometimes it doesn't quite feel—I guess nonbinary would be what I could potentially consider in the future. After some more therapy and self-examination and that type of thing. (*Tina, late 20s, cisgender woman*)

Jo, a genderqueer/nonbinary individual in their late 20s, described dysphoria more generally: "When I was younger, I experienced . . . a lot of stress and shame and self-hatred because of how my body looked, because of having PCOS." Other descriptions of shame or dysphoria attached to negative body image were more specifically evidenced in behaviors like the purposeful avoidance of reflective surfaces and mirrors, as shown by Farah and Josie:

Most of my negative feelings about my body are symptoms of PCOS . . . that I wish were different. I definitely have pretty negative views on my body, and just a lot of shame around how I look. My weight, my facial hair, I have a lot of shame about that, and embarrassment, just a lot of negative feelings. So, I . . . mostly avoid talking about it and thinking about it. And . . . I try not to examine myself too closely in a mirror. (*Farah, mid-20s, nonbinary*)

I still . . . base my whole worth off of what I look like. . . . And I try and avoid mirrors or reflective surfaces at all costs, and if I pass . . . a reflective surface or a mirror, I don't . . . look at it. (*Josie, early 20s, cisgender woman*)

Importantly, I found no published scientific literature that directly ties PCOS to dysphoria. Authors of one literature review concluded that prior research on PCOS does not support gender incongruence or dysphoria among those with PCOS, but that few studies have actually addressed this question directly (Liu et al., 2020). As illustrated by the interviews I conducted, negative body image and dysphoria appeared in narratives of both cisgender and gender diverse individuals. However, much future research is needed to discern the potential dysphoria resulting from PCOS bodies from that experienced by transgender individuals. As Julia Serano (2016) pointed out in her book on transsexuality, *Whipping Girl*, for trans people, violating appearance-related gender norms is secondary to the emotional pain of their felt gender not matching their physical sex. Whereas dysphoria may be a helpful frame for understanding body dissatisfaction experienced among cisgender individuals with PCOS, this dissatisfaction may not equate to the dissonance that reaches a threshold of emotional pain or debilitation for trans individuals.

Some individuals I interviewed, like Emerson, spoke of how an understanding of the transgender experience was helpful for their own process of coping with PCOS. Others highlighted how their experiences were similar in some ways to transmen and transwomen. Jules's experience with facial hair could actually be similar to those of trans*women* but overall described their experience in the "nebulous center" where a binary system for gender does not fit:

> I don't identify with . . . masculinity . . . at all. . . . But . . . in a weird way, . . . it's very . . . affirming to see that there are . . . people with PCOS that are transmen or are nonbinary. . . . They are having an experience with gender that is outside of . . . what would be expected. . . . And it may or may not be related to PCOS, but . . . in a weird way . . . that's . . . very . . . affirming to see. (*Emerson, mid-30s, nonbinary*)

> I find that with my own experience, because of my PCOS, I end up finding a lot of relation, like understanding with a lot of trans women. . . . [with] a lot of trans women that I have talked to . . . we've really been able to bond over the fact . . . that someone will look at you and misgender you immediately . . . as soon as they see a little stubble on your face. . . . I am kind of in this nebulous center area. . . . I feel so in the middle here and have the facial hair . . . with PCOS it is this very middle area . . . a lot of people consider being trans and transitioning to be very binary . . . transitioning from one to the other. . . . Whereas for me, it's like, I'm going from . . . dead center to . . . two degrees over. But I still consider myself trans and I'm still trans because I'm not female, and I was assigned female at birth. . . . I'm still working on my body image. . . . I'm going to be micro-dosing testosterone in order to actually enhance . . . my masculine features that I do want. But I do eventually plan on stopping testosterone and having my body be . . . at the medium I want it to be at, once I have achieved the permanent effect I want. . . . So, I'm more comfortable in my own body. . . . I have so many experiences that are similar and relatable . . . with both other transmen and transwomen . . . because while every trans experience is different, there really is no such thing as a binary trans experience. . . . not that there's not binary trans people, but . . . gender in general is not strictly binary. (*Jules, late 20s, nonbinary*)

Despite symptoms of PCOS that violate gendered norms, half of those I interviewed identified their gender as female, and many described within their narratives their journeys of coming to some level of acceptance that womanhood must not be defined so rigidly. Kim described this journey as coming to accept the variety of ways women can present, including with facial and body hair. Similarly, Alia, after perceiving her body was losing femininity due to the masculinizing traits of PCOS, described the identity-related journey as coming to accept womanhood as fluid:

> I . . . feel pretty clear that I'm a woman. I don't think I've ever really had to question my gender identity. . . . I think the way that I perform my gender looks different than the ways that I grew up being taught women are supposed to be . . . because there are physical characteristics, like having facial hair or

beard, that are really strongly associated with . . . men . . . has made me think at times . . . I shouldn't . . . have hair on my chin because I'm a woman, . . . but over time, I've gotten more comfortable saying that . . . some women have beards and mustaches and that's . . . the variety of . . . human experience. It wasn't . . . always like that, though . . . I struggled a lot more with gender identity and presentation when I was younger and . . . fitting more rigid gender identity when I was younger. . . . I feel a little more comfortable with the fluidity and less binary, even though I identify as a woman. I don't maybe feel the need to present in that very binary way. (*Kim, mid-30s, cisgender woman*)

[PCOS] really did affect my view of who I was in my identity in terms of my gender, because my body started to change. . . . I was growing hair on my face. . . . I was gaining so much weight and my body was kind of losing some of its femininity in my mind. And then I started to wonder . . . is this who I am? What does that mean? My physicality—how much does that affect my gender identity? . . . I really did have these moments of wondering where did I fit . . . PCOS—because of the physical effects on my body, I definitely felt . . . very confused. But over time and talking and—and getting to know people, I really also began to understand that the word woman . . . means something—it means something to me . . . I realized that . . . I do fit in with the gender identity, a woman and a female. This condition . . . happening to me due to hereditary reasons . . . doesn't just magically take something away . . . I always felt female. I never really felt not female just because people were putting things on to me. So . . . even though I had a huge period of confusion, I . . . came back to myself being female. But it's . . . with great respect to fluidity, because the truth is that this idea of what a woman is . . . maybe it's more fluid than we think it is. And basically, even though . . . my mind is a bit more open because of PCOS, I still do think I am female. (*Alia, early 30s, cisgender woman*)

BREAKING NEW GROUND: POSITIVE PCOS EXPERIENCES AMONG THE GENDER DIVERSE

To summarize thus far, we have considered that symptoms of PCOS violate societal expectations for female bodies, thereby threatening womanhood and contributing to negative body image or even dysphoria in both cisgender women and gender diverse individuals living with PCOS. Next, let us consider the possibility that for some, PCOS symptoms are less negative and even welcomed characteristics. The remainder of the chapter explores how PCOS may be experienced differently by those whose identities are gender diverse.

This section of the chapter expands what we had previously known about the experience of PCOS, which has been limited to cisgender women's experiences through the lens of binary gender. In the preface, I briefly defined gender-related terms. Let us return to some of those terms, this time with deeper explanation, to ensure a solid foundation on which to build the remainder of the chapter focused on gender diversity. Specifically, let us expand on the gender terms *sex*, *gender*, and the *gender binary*. For years, I taught students in my undergraduate-level Psychology of Women course that the difference between sex and gender was biology; sex was about biology and being male or female, whereas gender was about the social identity and characteristics society attaches to being a man or a woman. I emphasized, as a "good feminist" would, that this means that the traits commonly associated with being a woman were not biologically determined but rather culturally based through the process of socialization (see Fausto-Sterling, 2019, for additional reading on the evolution of this distinction). Judith Butler, (1990) in her book *Gender Trouble*, questions this distinction, arguing that sex itself could be culturally constructed; our gendered culture is the context in which sex differentiation is determined. Other recent scholars in this area have convincingly argued that sex and gender (i.e., biology and socialization) are intricately linked and use the term *gender/sex* to acknowledge that sex and gender cannot easily be disentangled (Fausto-Sterling, 2019; van Anders, 2015). This inextricable link between sex (the biological body) and gender (the social experience) are evident in the excerpts from gender diverse individuals living with PCOS described in this section.

In addition, the limitations of trying to distinguish sex from gender make clear that the typical use of the terms sex and gender actually perpetuates a sex and gender binary system that does not account for the full spectrum of lived experiences of sex and gender. Although trans individuals can fit within a binary system of gender, such as when individuals assigned male at birth self-identify as women or individuals assigned female at birth self-identify as men, not all individuals fit this binary. An entire group of people identify their gender as outside of the binary system and may self-identify with labels, such as nonbinary, genderfluid, or genderqueer. Thus, individuals who identify as nonbinary call into question the gender binary system, a system called further into question by scholars who have documented empirical findings from neuroscience, behavioral endocrinology, psychological research, and developmental research that challenge the gender binary (Hyde et al., 2019). Furthermore, the commonly used terms *cisgender* and *transgender* actually refer to a binary of gender that either matches or does not match sex assigned at birth and leave out those born intersex, given that their sex does not fit a male–female binary (Viloria & Nieto, 2020). The very fact that intersex people exist makes the binary system obsolete. Our current system of identification limits understanding of the complexity of lived experiences of gender/sex. These limitations apply to what is known and unknown about PCOS experience, as you will see here.

Concordance Between PCOS and Gender Identity

Although symptoms of PCOS can indeed be stigmatizing for their violation of gender-based societal expectations, for some, PCOS symptoms may actually align with gender identity. Whereas threatened womanhood, negative body image, and dysphoria appeared to stem from a dissonance between expectations for female bodies and the reality of bodies, some individuals with PCOS may identify less strongly with female bodies or womanhood. In fact, a subgroup of those with PCOS do not identify as women at all and therefore may not evaluate themselves against feminine standards. As a result, these individuals may experience less distress when their bodies defy the expectations for women or female bodies—and may even experience positivity due to PCOS defying traditional conceptions of gender. This possibility may help to explain the one finding in published research on transgender men, showing less gender dysphoria and less negative body image in trans men with PCOS than those without PCOS (Gezer et al., 2021).

In an illustrative excerpt, Riley described how identifying as nonbinary changed the lived experience of masculine characteristics of PCOS from feelings of shame to those of neutrality. In the second excerpt, Riley clarified that bodily nonconformity to expectations resulting from PCOS can even feel affirming:

> Some of the characteristics . . . that you get with PCOS . . . are usually associated more with . . . male secondary sex characteristics. I guess a lot of them used to make me feel really bad because I felt like . . . I wasn't even allowed the choice to . . . conform to the standards that society placed on women, but . . . now that I . . . felt more neutral about it and have realized that I'm nonbinary, they don't bother me as much. . . . I guess I moved from kind of shame about some more traditionally masculine qualities to just kind of viewing it neutrally. (*Riley, early 20s, nonbinary*)

> Sometimes I do want to . . . be very feminine, but my PCOS doesn't really get in the way of that anymore, at least in my viewpoint. I don't feel like it gets in the way of that anymore. . . . Before . . . I knew I was nonbinary . . . I definitely felt like a girl but like . . . society said . . . I wasn't conforming to being a girl in some of the ways I was expected to and some of those ways weren't even possible for me because of . . . how my hormones played out. . . . I gave it a lot of thought and now that I kind of view it more neutrally, it can sometimes be even a little affirming to not conform to what a woman is supposed to be or what not. (*Riley, early 20s, nonbinary*)

Individuals with gender diverse identities experienced specific symptoms of PCOS, such as irregular menstrual periods, positively. Menstruation is associated with womanhood, and therefore individuals assigned female at birth who have diverse (e.g., masculine) gender identities may have negative attitudes about it because of the continual reminders that their bodies do not match with their identity (Chrisler et al., 2016). Some individuals with PCOS who identified their gender identity in more masculine ways, such as Marsh, welcomed the lack of menstruation common to the experience of PCOS. Others, such as Ricky, additionally chose hormone therapy to suppress their menstrual cycle and bring about more masculine features.

> I decided I really didn't like having periods and didn't want them again, which probably is related to gender identity. I always felt like that was a great symptom of PCOS, that I enjoyed not having periods. . . . I've never had pain, pelvic pain. . . . I've never really had any of the very unpleasant kind of symptoms of this. I've mostly just had things that suit my gender identity and things that are just convenient, like not having a period. . . . And so, I'm sort of a weird case where I feel like PCOS has been just mostly beneficial to me. (*Marsh, mid-30s, nonbinary*)

> I take testosterone now. I started that when I was 31, so it's been 10 years and I don't have periods usually. They do happen every once in a while, but I don't usually have them usually. But the whole system sort of seems dormant or shut down. So, I don't have any pain either. Usually. (*Ricky, early 40s, nonbinary*)

Individuals with gender diverse identities also perceived hirsutism positively. As discussed in Chapter 1, many individuals with PCOS have signs of hyperandrogenism or more androgens (e.g., testosterone) than typical females, causing features like excess or male-patterned body hair (also called hirsutism). Whereas the first half of this chapter described how excess hair is strongly linked with masculinity and threatened womanhood, for some individuals with PCOS, the masculinizing body or facial hair may bring acceptance. For this subset of individuals with PCOS, male-patterned body hair actually corresponds with their gender identity as nonbinary, trans, or genderfluid. Frederick, who identified as a man in his early 20s, concluded: "For a lot of people with PCOS, they do see a man in the mirror. But it's about whether you're okay with that or whether you're not."

PCOS as Asset (or "Superpower") for Diverse Gender Identity

Not only can gender diverse identity correspond with PCOS symptoms, some symptoms of PCOS may actually be considered an asset *because* they are masculinizing. Kendall, a nonbinary individual in their early 20s, summed it up by saying that "with PCOS, it's made my appearance a lot more what I was looking for anyways."

The symptom of hirsutism, in particular, may provide an advantage to individuals who are trans or nonbinary who strive to look masculine. Jonny just started taking testosterone and described the advantage of increased body hair due to PCOS. Marsh, who was on testosterone for a year, described the masculinizing advantage due to PCOS as a "blessing" and acknowledged how such positive experience attached to increased hair is different from those who want to look feminine:

> I've been taking testosterone . . . for a little over a month. And . . . in one way . . . I'm a step ahead of—of the people that are just starting testosterone or even some people that have been on it for a couple of years. Because I already have facial hair. I already have chest hair. (*Jonny, early 30s, nonbinary/transmasc*)

> I actually think it's a blessing ultimately for me that I had sort of a head start with some of the changes that have made me feel more comfortable in my body, as far as testosterone goes. So, I think for a lot of people, especially people who are women and . . . identify as more feminine and want to look more feminine, this is a struggle for them because their bodies are sort of betraying them with body hair and things that are perceived as masculine that they don't want. For me, it's been a blessing, because I already had more facial hair than most people do on several years of testosterone. I, my hairline had started changing when I went off of estrogen birth control and had an IUD for a few years. And I didn't realize it. I kind of "woke up" in the middle of already being a few years into a low dose of transition, just because my body was doing it. My body took to androgen very well. I've been on testosterone just a little over a year and I have a full beard. And a lot of these changes, a lot of other like trans masculine people really struggle to get and to achieve. And they just happened so fast for me because my body was sort of tuned to it already. So, I feel like that's been a blessing for me. (*Marsh, mid-30s, nonbinary*)

This masculinizing advantage due to PCOS may be noticed by others and seen as a source of envy by transgender friends because PCOS naturally engenders bodily features that others can bring about only through hormone therapy. Jo described the ability to have facial and body hair without taking testosterone as a "superpower" and further described it as celebrated in trans spaces:

> When I'm in trans spaces, it's sort of seen as something that's celebrated. Like I've had a lot of trans guys asked me if I'm on testosterone because normally people don't have the amount of facial and body hair that I have until they go on testosterone for a couple years. And so, it feels like a really cool thing that I'm able to look this way without that. (*Jo, late 20s, genderqueer/nonbinary*)

In addition to hirsutism, menstrual irregularities and masculine body shape can make life better for those who are gender diverse. Jonny further described having these symptoms as helpful because it can avoid the dysphoria many experience when they have menstrual cycles:

> I feel like specifically for trans people that have PCOS—at face value . . . it is helpful. Because . . . some people get dysphoria from having their—their cycle.

And [with PCOS] you have a lessened amount of cycles or it doesn't come as often . . . it . . . can give you . . . the typical male pattern . . . [of] hair growth. . . . And so . . . that could be perceived as . . . helpful. . . . and then also . . . the body shape as well. . . . if you have a more masculine shape to begin with then you're already ahead of the game. (*Jonny, early 30s, nonbinary/transmasc*)

Importantly, however, any positive experiences attached to particular PCOS symptoms were balanced with negative PCOS encounters, both before and after identification as trans, nonbinary, or otherwise gender diverse.

But the gender dysphoria, like I feel like PCOS actually helps a little bit. But it also kind of makes it worse because I'm having all these problems that revolve around my female anatomy. So it's kind of like a push and pull of two differing emotions. . . . And before I felt as though I was ready to identify as transgender, it definitely made me feel terrible about my body, very much like I was unlikable, unattractive to other people, but now I feel the opposite. I feel like it makes me more attractive because I'm transgender now and I present masculinely. But at the same time the health aspects and if I don't watch myself, I could gain weight. Then I will feel even worse about myself. (*Kendall, early 20s, nonbinary*)

COMPLEX QUESTIONS REMAIN ABOUT THE LINKS BETWEEN PCOS AND GENDER IDENTITY

Thus far, this chapter has outlined (a) the negative experiences of those with PCOS who encounter threatened womanhood, negative body image, or even dysphoria due to PCOS violating gender-related expectations and (b) the positive experiences of PCOS symptoms, such as hirsutism and irregular menstruation, reported among individuals with diverse gender identities due to their correspondence with nonbinary or transgender identities. Whereas the first set of findings supported prior research on PCOS, the second set contributes new information on an understudied subset of the PCOS population. However, more research is urgently needed on gender diversity in PCOS. In fact, differences in experience of PCOS symptoms by gender identification discussed in this chapter highlight some specific underexamined questions I would like to explore in the remainder of the chapter. These compelling questions have little to no psychological research examining them thus far.

Is There a Link Between PCOS and Diverse Gender Identity?

This first unresolved question raised by those I interviewed addresses the possible linkage between PCOS and gender identity, as illustrated by Tracy:

> I'm just so used to being . . . very androgynous . . . some people . . . had to transition or . . . realize that they're nonbinary. . . . I . . . also had to realize I was nonbinary, but mostly because I didn't know the term, not because I . . . had to realize something about myself. . . . I . . . feel very much like this has always been . . . who I am . . . I wondered if that's the result of having PCOS . . . and like what would be the case if I didn't? (*Tracy, early 30s, nonbinary*)

So far, this question has been explored either by recruiting those with PCOS and asking about gender identity or recruiting gender diverse individuals and asking about PCOS. Limited research has taken the first strategy to examine diverse gender identity in individuals with PCOS compared with control individuals without PCOS. In one study conducted in Poland, those with PCOS over age 30 reported more severe hirsutism and saw themselves as sexually undifferentiated and more androgynous (e.g., Kowalczyk et al., 2012). Similarly, limited research on gender diverse individuals has examined whether they have PCOS. In a Japanese study that examined the medical cases of 238 female-to-male transsexual patients who presented at a gender identity disorder clinic, researchers found that of those who had never received hormone therapy ($n = 128$), 32% had diagnosable PCOS according to the Rotterdam criteria (Baba et al., 2011). In a study of transsexuals in Serbia, researchers reported that 14.4% of the female-to-male transsexuals had PCOS according to Rotterdam criteria (Vujovic et al., 2009). Although both of these estimates are greater than general prevalence rates of PCOS reported in Chapter 1, these rates are difficult to interpret given the limitations of their sampling strategies and the lack of representative studies examining PCOS.

We can neither confirm nor deny a link between PCOS and gender identity when such limited information exists about PCOS in gender diverse individuals and vice versa. Within the narratives of individuals with PCOS whom I interviewed, there was what appeared to be an inextricable link between PCOS traits and their identification. To be clear, no one claimed that PCOS caused them to identify as trans, nonbinary, or otherwise gender diverse. Rather, the masculinizing traits experienced with PCOS seemed to contribute to their perceptions of themselves and were confounded with gender identification processes. As illustrated by Frederick's excerpt, with PCOS, individuals already see masculine features in the mirror, whereas others may just wish they saw them:

> I grew up . . . seeing my male traits, and I believe that is . . . intertwined with my male identity and trans identity. Because it [PCOS] didn't show up, of course, until puberty . . . I was assigned female at birth. But then I show up with these male traits later in life, seeing a male in the mirror, because I have male traits and I feel like it's possible if I didn't have those male traits, I may not be trans. There's no way of me knowing. So . . . my experience is very different

from people who don't have like PCOS or other conditions like that, because they usually grow up looking in a mirror and wanting to be a man, not seeing male traits or a man. (*Frederick, early 20s, man*)

Similarly, Rory described how not meeting expectations for gender created a flexibility in thinking about gender, clarifying further that PCOS did not create that process but rather shaped or supported the process of coming to a nonbinary gender identity. Ellis also mentioned a more recent recognition that PCOS permitted an exploration of gender identity due to violating the societal assumption that being a woman means menstruating. For Kendall, PCOS seemed to help with gender transitioning through greater body acceptance.

PCOS, for me, has . . . led me to points where I was able to . . . challenge my own . . . gender identity. Not saying that specifically . . . PCOS . . . made me . . . queer or trans . . . but . . . opening up more questions about . . . my gender as a whole, just because my body wasn't fully fitting into this. And so . . . once my body wasn't fully fitting into things, . . . it just allowed me question other things that just weren't fitting together. And as I became more aware of . . . different options for gender and that . . . I could be . . . nonbinary—I really didn't have to be like a cis woman . . . something felt right. . . . I think PCOS is definitely . . . not creating that process, but it shaped that process because it definitely . . . allowed me to ask more questions than I think I would've if my body was so regularly accepted within . . . the cis . . . female schema. (*Rory, early 20s, nonbinary*)

Part of the reason I have always felt . . . not attached to being female or a girl . . . is because I don't have a period. Because . . . one thing that is always touted . . . having a period, it makes you a girl. Having a period makes you a woman. . . . And I was like, "OK, well, none of this applies to me, so it doesn't matter anymore." And so, I realized that gender wasn't something that I had to confine myself to, because I never really fit in the box to begin with. And then, not having a period, "OK, well, I'm not a girl anyway, so who cares?" But that's only something that I realized recently . . . that being diagnosed with PCOS allowed me to explore my gender identity more. (*Ellis, mid-20s, nonbinary*)

I feel like even if I didn't have PCOS [I] still had ended up trans anyways, but it definitely helped me come to terms with my body and just love the body that I was in. And it helped the transition go a lot smoother, I believe. (*Kendall, early 20s, nonbinary*)

Importantly, however, when individuals discussed a connection between PCOS and diverse gender identity, there was an acknowledgment that not everyone with PCOS identifies as gender diverse. Having PCOS does not equate to having diverse gender identification, as illustrated by Jules, a nonbinary individual with PCOS in their late 20s, "There's a lot of cis women out there who . . . have PCOS and that doesn't change their gender identity."

As such, rather than a specific statement on the relationship between PCOS and gender identity, the main conclusions I draw from the positive PCOS experiences among gender diverse individuals are (a) recognizing that not all individuals living with PCOS identify as cisgender women and (b) individual experience of PCOS symptoms may vary by gender identity.

Is PCOS an Intersex Condition?

Another unresolved—and quite frankly, controversial—question about PCOS is whether it can be considered an intersex condition. Admittedly, tackling this question adequately in the context of this book is daunting. Although I have studied the LGBTQ experience of stigma and health for more than a decade, little of that work has crossed into the realm of intersex classification. Why, then, am I bringing up this topic at all? In my interviews, some individuals reported that the question of PCOS as an intersex condition was coming up in PCOS circles. For example, Alia described becoming aware of PCOS as a possible intersex condition through online support group discussions. Leah described learning about the possibility during a training she had completed as part of her job, as well as the same online support group. Thus, I felt compelled to investigate the intersex classification and explore how PCOS may or may not fit within it.

> I am a member of PCOS groups online and something that has come up in discussions, is the idea of . . . does testosterone—having a high level—does that mean you're part of the intersex community, because you have both male and female attributes? . . . And that made me kind of wonder, like, do I have both male and female parts of me? Am I maybe not quite one or the other? (*Alia, early 30s, cisgender woman*)

Leah, a cisgender woman(ish) in her mid-40s, said that "they talked about PCOS as an intersex condition, which it really is . . . you have so much more androgens. So, it does sort of change . . . your sex in some ways."

In my investigation, I read published articles on intersex classification as well as popular books and memoirs to understand both the more medicalized viewpoints and the lived perspectives of those who are intersex. Because this work has afforded me an introductory understanding of the history of the term *intersex* and an appreciation for the reality that any sex classification system is embedded in sociocultural context, a full critique of the cultural context in which we classify sex is beyond the scope of this book. Instead, I focus on key points that might explain why individuals with PCOS might perceive it to be an intersex condition and clarify the controversy over naming PCOS as an intersex condition.

Before outlining these key points, it is necessary to clarify the term; *intersex* is an umbrella term that refers to having biological sex characteristics that differ from those typically associated with males or females. However, not everyone agrees with the use of this term. In fact, the official term currently used in medical settings is disorders of sex development (DSD), which refers to atypical chromosomal, gonadal, and anatomic sex due to congenital conditions, and was determined at the 2005 Chicago Consensus Meeting (Lee et al., 2006). A surface-level comparison of these two terms—intersex versus DSD—can illustrate part of the history to which I refer. Whereas DSD considers variation in sex as disordered and genetically based, intersex references sex as broader human variation rather than a strict or genetically based system and is, unsurprisingly, less stigmatizing and preferred by many intersex individuals and activists (e.g., Griffiths, 2018). For more consideration of this topic from an intersex perspective, I recommend reading Hil Malatino's (2019) *Queer Embodiment* and Hida Viloria's (2017) *Born Both*.

What is it about PCOS that would make some view it as an intersex condition? My understanding of the argument in favor of PCOS as an intersex condition is that PCOS symptoms could also be classified as secondary sex characteristics. PCOS symptoms often include excess testosterone for what might be typically associated with being female, creating excess and male-patterned body and facial hair, for instance. Similarly, some with PCOS experience male-patterned baldness or hair thinning or more masculine body shape. Additionally, irregular or missing periods or anovulation is a common symptom. Given these bodily characteristics related to increased testosterone, higher levels of which are typically associated with being male, an argument might be made for PCOS as a form of intersex—or broad variation in sex characteristics typical for males or females.

Although less technical but perhaps persuasive, some individuals I interviewed described feeling validated by the term intersex to describe PCOS experiences. Some even self-identified as intersex. For example, Jules self-identified as intersex and described the positive impact that the revelation of PCOS as a possible intersex condition had. Jules further described how intersex self-identification can validate hormonal variation and masculine secondary sex characteristics with PCOS that are seen as abnormal for females:

> One of the biggest revelations for me . . . was finding out that PCOS . . . in its way, can be considered a form of being intersex. And that just—it blew me away. And honestly, that's something that I think is almost revolutionary and mind-blowing in scope, because . . . that helped me so much and . . . helped me get society into perspective in a way as well. (*Jules, late 20s, nonbinary*)

When I learned the connection of PCOS and intersex, it just was so incredibly validating and it really helped me embrace myself. It's one of the reasons why one of my primary identities, when asked how I identify, I will always mention intersex because I really think it's important as well, for people to understand how commonplace it is to not be born in what people think is the normal gender binary. . . . I almost feel like living proof that you cannot box up sex or gender . . . because we are each who we are. . . . I am biologically me—my biology is unique to myself. I was never biologically male nor female, but yet I was never medically acknowledged intersex. I was medically acknowledged as a freak. . . . So, I think that's really something that needs to come into the mainstream as well, where it's like all of our hormones are different. (*Jules, late 20s, nonbinary*)

Considering PCOS in relation to intersex appeared to help individuals make sense of their PCOS bodies and experiences. Marsh described how coming to an intersex self-identification made sense in light of being "in between" many identities, whether gender, racial/ethnic, or sexual:

So, at this point, it's [PCOS] . . . another part of me and who I am and . . . it's . . . weirdly an important part of me, because it's this diagnosis that has changed my body significantly and impacted my way of walking through the world. But it's not . . . a negative diagnosis to me. It's been sort of like . . . an identity. I really think that it's accepting that it's . . . considered intersex and . . . realizing that it's part of being somewhere "in between" [that] really helped me, because I'm somewhere between races, I'm somewhere in between sexuality, I'm not straight or gay, I'm not [one racial/ethnic identity] or [second racial/ethnic identity]. . . . I'm just like in-between so many things. . . . It just felt like . . . I'm biracial, bisexual—of course, I'm also intersex. . . . It just feels like "of course I'm in between everything." (*Marsh, mid-30s, nonbinary*)

Jo expressed, quite compellingly, a similar validation attached to an intersex identity because neither their PCOS body nor gender identity fits with their assigned sex. Despite reporting mixed emotions about the challenges attached to violating societal expectations of gender, Jo further described *leaning in* to "a sort of freakishness that feels kind of authentic":

The more I've let go of the need to think of myself as female and perform femininity or womanhood in any kind of culturally defined way, I've . . . come to see myself as . . . an anomalous body . . . my body doesn't make sense in terms of sex or gender to most people, because we . . . have a system where people will only treat you as a person if they can legibly read your gender and then fit you into a gendered box. And that's hard for people to do that to me, both because of my physical characteristics and my gender presentation, and that's definitely affected by PCOS. And sometimes that's terrible. And I hate how it makes me feel, but most of time I kind of just lean into this sort of freakishness and that feels kind of authentic, and . . . almost appealing, because I don't have to lie and . . . I can embrace the differences that my body has. And I think that feels like an important part of my gender nonconforming identity because at this point it feels like it would be so much more work to live my life and make myself appear as my assigned gender, which is part of the reason why I think it makes more sense for me to think of myself as intersex rather than as a female assigned person who is trans or . . . a woman with a hormonal condition. And so, I guess that's complicated, because that's good and bad at the same time. At this point, it's mostly good. It is something that feels really . . . uniquely authentic about myself and my experience. And that's . . . how I've come to understand my own transness . . . neither my body nor my gender fits the category that I was assigned to. (*Jo, late 20s, genderqueer/nonbinary*)

This validation was quite emotional for some who have searched for understanding about their own experiences of PCOS, as illustrated by Emerson, whose tears during our interview when discussing the topic of intersex reflected a sense of relief about herself:

But . . . it has really helped me that there—there is a community of people who feel like PCOS is an intersex condition. And that's a journey that I've been on lately. And that has really, really help how I feel about myself. And just knowing . . . even though . . . I don't identify with like masculinity . . . at all. . . . it's very . . . affirming to see that there are a lot of people with PCOS that are transmen or are nonbinary. And like they are having an experience with gender that is outside of . . . what would be expected. And it may or may not be related to PCOS, but like in a weird way . . . it's very like affirming to see that . . . I'm sorry that I'm crying like, but it's not really in a sad way. Like, it's just—this is very personal right now because something that I've been experiencing very recently. But it's been really great. (*Emerson, mid-30s, nonbinary*)

Despite these lived experiences of those with PCOS who appear to embrace an intersex identity, at least at the time of writing this book, I found no published literature to indicate that PCOS is an intersex condition. Given the lack of discussion surrounding the possible link between PCOS and intersex, I am forced to assume that the explanation lies in the fact that the medical classification of intersex (DSD) is based on genetic and chromosomal differences rather than hormonal ones that would include PCOS. Indeed, DSD typically refers to individuals who have atypical or ambiguous genitalia that also are often noticed upon birth or in childhood, although later presentation in adolescence or adulthood is possible (e.g., P. A. Lee et al., 2016). In contrast, PCOS involves increased testosterone, which translates into secondary sex characteristics that are masculinizing, and, according to the limited published literature on the topic, these apparently are not enough to call into question classification as female. In his book on PCOS, Samuel Thatcher (2000) wrote: "Those with PCOS should not be alarmed if told that your male hormones are elevated; be assured that you are completely female" (p. 19). Importantly, whereas this statement may validate some, others may find validation within the self-identification of intersex.

An important acknowledgment when discussing the intersex community is that many intersex individuals have experienced severely traumatic medical treatments beginning at birth. If you are unfamiliar with this literature that includes memoirs of personal experiences of intersex individuals, I encourage further reading. Considering this point, entertaining the possibility of PCOS as intersex may be seen as diminishing the experiences of intersex individuals. This caveat was referenced in the interviews I conducted. Emerson acknowledged that the experience of PCOS may not present the difficulties that individuals otherwise intersex commonly encounter, such as unwanted surgeries:

> I would never want to be . . . super loud about it and take away from people who have had . . . medical trauma that they didn't consent to from . . . a very young age. . . . I would never want to do that. But . . . a good part of the intersex community is very welcoming to people with PCOS. And . . . that's really awesome . . . I've definitely seen a lot more of that than . . . gatekeeping or "you're not intersex enough unless . . . you had surgery against your will when you were . . . born or when you were . . . five" . . . so . . . that's been really cool. (*Emerson, mid-30s, nonbinary*)

In sum, PCOS has not been formally considered within the intersex classification. In fact, I could find no published works that even discuss the possibility. Yet reports of individuals I interviewed indicated that the term as a self-identification can be helpful for explaining symptoms of PCOS that may complicate their self-perceptions of sex and gender. Statements made by the medical community presumably intended to assure women with PCOS that they are female despite the increased androgens may be invalidating for a subgroup of those with PCOS. The current view that PCOS in not an intersex condition appears to be based solely on a medicalized intersex classification that, as some have written, does not consider the cultural context and psychosocial impact of living in a body that does not fit within normative expectations for females (e.g., Griffiths, 2018). At the very least, this chapter evidences that both PCOS and intersex tend to be perceived by the medical community as abnormal and needing professional intervention to align the body with societal expectations for sex and gender. Similar to Hil Malatino's (2019) perspective in *Queer Embodiment*, we might benefit from challenging our assumptions that bodies (whether PCOS or intersex) are "errors" or "failures" that need to be changed if individuals with these bodies are happy with them.

CONCLUSION: GENDER TRANSGRESSIONS AND TRANSGRESSING GENDER

In this chapter, I presented evidence for a gendered embodiment of PCOS, or that personal experience with PCOS symptoms may depend on correspondence between gender-related expectations and one's gender identity. This chapter broke new ground by presenting diverse gender experiences in PCOS—experiences that need more attention, as Jean noted:

> There are diverse experiences of PCOS . . . PCOS is not just something that's impacting cis women. There are trans people who have PCOS or intersex people who have PCOS, like making space for them to be part of the conversation too, and all of those different experiences. (*Jean, late 20s, cisgender woman*)

Much more psychological research is needed on the gendered embodiment of PCOS. This research should consider the complexity of defining sex and gender, the limitations of the gender binary, and the restrictive expectations based on them. As shown in this chapter, there are painful consequences to having such restrictive expectations for female bodies. Perhaps moving beyond counting the gender transgressions brought on by PCOS symptoms, we as a community of scholars, advocates, and individuals with PCOS might consider ways to intentionally transgress our outdated notions of sex and gender to allow for more flexible ways of being. In the next chapter, I explore how social support and close relationships might be impacted by PCOS or its symptoms, which can be stigmatizing based on one's gendered embodiment, as has been shown in Chapters 2 and 3.

4 SOCIAL SUPPORT AND CLOSE RELATIONSHIPS IN THE PCOS CONTEXT

Until I could face the truth, I had my secret, and my secret had me.
—Dr. Edith Eger (2020, p. 75), *The Gift: 12 Lessons to Save Your Life*

This fourth chapter of the book describes ways in which polycystic ovary syndrome (PCOS) might influence elements of close relationships. Typically, close relationships involve those with mutual influence or some emotional bond, such as friendships, partners, family, and the like (Duggan, 2019). This means that formal relationships, such as those with professionals like health care providers or employers, would fall outside of the realm of close relationships. Additionally, whereas individuals might be able to describe how large their network of close relationships is and the extent of their integration within it, this chapter rather deals with the content of those close relationships (House et al., 1988). For example, rather than how many friends and family members individuals have, this chapter considers the availability and experiences of social support from friends, family, and community. Although prior research has focused on the impact that physical illness can have

https://doi.org/10.1037/0000337-005
The Psychology of PCOS: Building the Science and Breaking the Silence, by S. L. Williams

on the content of close personal relationships (Duggan, 2019), none of that work has ever been applied to understanding close relationships in PCOS. Thus, I describe the close relationship processes that the individuals whom I interviewed suggested as relevant in their PCOS experience. The two main sections of this chapter cover (a) social support and related processes and (b) experiences with sexuality and relationship partners and dating.

SOCIAL SUPPORT AND RELATED PROCESSES IN PCOS

We know without a doubt that human beings are social animals and that close relationships with others are important to us. One of the reasons relationships are important is for the social support they provide. Availability of social support can influence our health (Cohen et al., 2000). For example, when we have support available to us during times of need, we can be protected from some of the harmful effects that stressful experiences might otherwise have on our mental and physical health (Schwarzer & Leppin, 1991). However, social support is not an endless resource. In fact, it can erode due to life circumstances (Barrera, 1986), and we might find ourselves wishing we had more social support and connection. Further, sometimes the reality of our social lives is that even though social support network members, such as family members, are available, their offers of support may not *feel* supportive.

Lack of PCOS Support

You might be surprised to learn that individuals experiencing a common physical condition that affects millions of individuals across the United States and the globe report a lack of PCOS-specific social support. Individuals whom I interviewed consistently reported a lack of social support in their lives, particularly in relation to PCOS. Some of this missing support appeared attributable to behaviors of close others, such as family, who put pressure on them to change their physical appearance to fit into societal norms, particularly about femininity. Additionally, some chose not to disclose their PCOS or avoided particular social situations, possibly due to a perceived lack of support. Regardless of its evolution, however, this lack of social support is unfortunate given the context of PCOS, which can be stigmatizing and stressful—the very context in which social support might be most beneficial. Yet some individuals reported positive social experiences emerging out of PCOS and felt social support in their lives. These supportive encounters typically occurred when they were interacting with like others who also had PCOS.

To the extent that we consider PCOS a stigmatized condition, lack of support is less surprising. Fewer available support resources have been reported among individuals with other stigmatized characteristics, whether due to the ways that others treat them for their stigma or the ways they feel about themselves and choose to conceal their stigma (e.g., Hatzenbuehler et al., 2009). The overall invisibility of PCOS in society may further exacerbate the social support problem as well; network members may not know that social support is needed for the health condition. Feelings of misunderstanding within the narratives were similar to previous reports by individuals with PCOS who felt isolated and that no one understood them (Wright et al., 2020). An illustrative excerpt comes from my interview with Amy, who referenced a lack of understanding from close others, including friends, family, and partners:

> Some of my . . . friends are not as understanding and sometimes my family might not be, as well. My . . . ex did not really understand why sometimes . . . I couldn't do the things that she wanted me to do, especially if it was like a bad day and I was in a lot of pain. She . . . always said that she understood but you could tell that her understanding was . . . conditional because she didn't have to experience it. And, so, it kind of put a strain on the relationship. . . . And the depression comes with its own . . . stigma and that that's another thing that people can't really wrap their head around unless they have experienced something similar or they know somebody that's gone through it. . . . I don't think that a lot of people understand that depression is more than just sadness. (*Amy, mid-20s, cisgender woman*)

This lack of understanding may be tied to the larger problem of invisibility of PCOS, which those with the condition explicitly mentioned. Because of invisibility, people likely do not know what PCOS is and therefore what those with PCOS go through. In fact, invisibility presented as one of the hardest things about having PCOS, according to those I interviewed, such as Amethyst:

> I feel like the hardest thing is people not understanding what it is . . . you're trying to explain to someone how you feel, they don't understand because it's not something that people widely know about and people don't hear about. So, they don't really understand. (*Amethyst, mid-20s, cisgender woman*)

Lack of PCOS-specific support was also represented in reports of inadequate community support. Leah, for instance, described how helpful it would be to have a community to know that people with PCOS live past 30, implying the lack of community she felt for her age group in particular. Loren explicitly contrasted the helpfulness of having the community attached to cultural or ethnic identity and not feeling that same sense of community with PCOS.

> When I was . . . 18 and first getting diagnosed . . . I think it would have been helpful to have . . . a community and a sense of . . . what older people with PCOS . . . are going through and that they have community, and that they don't all just die at 30. (*Leah, mid-40s, cisgender(ish) woman*)

> I'm [racial/ethnic identity] and people assigned female at birth that are [racial/ethnic identity] usually have a lot of hair and the body hair is usually dark and thick . . . that has made things slightly better in that I know people even who don't have PCOS who also struggle with the body hair situation, where it's just kind of like, oh, that's our culture. We all have super thick leg hair . . . get our face waxed, that sort of thing. So, I've seen . . . body positivity over . . . thick and dark body hair. So, I think that has helped a bit of having that cultural community, because I don't feel PCOS community. (*Loren, early 20s, nonbinary*)

This finding of lacking community may be understood by considering prior work on stigma too, where some stigmatized characteristics (e.g., minoritized race/ethnicity) were associated with strong group identity and community, whereas others were not (e.g., obesity; see Major et al., 2012). The lack of felt community in individuals with PCOS may show that they may not feel like an identity group as members of racial/ethnic or gender identity groups do. Feeling a lack of community support in PCOS may also reflect the reality of limited access to a PCOS community. Although online PCOS support communities do exist on social media sites like Facebook, the social support appeared not to fit everyone's needs equally. Jean highlighted the diversity of the syndrome itself and how vastly different the issues people struggle with are, posing problems for feeling supported in these communities:

> When I first got diagnosed, I remember . . . looking for spaces to try and process it . . . they just weren't spaces that really fit my experience. And, so, I ended up joining this Facebook group that somebody else had made specifically for queer people who have PCOS. And . . . it's fine. But . . . a lot of the issues that people are talking . . . about are the issues that aren't the most significant to me. And the issues that are significant to me . . . are less serious or less fixable. So, I just kind of feel like I'm stuck. And . . . I just feel like . . . when I talk to people that I already knew personally who have PCOS, our experiences of it are very different. (*Jean, late 20s, cisgender woman*)

Lack of support felt in these online PCOS communities appeared heightened for individuals with diverse gender identities. Absence of support may be salient for nonbinary individuals, for example, because support resources are biased toward cisgender women, especially given the woman-centered language surrounding who is impacted by PCOS. This lack of support due to the invisibility of gender diversity in PCOS was illustrated by Riley, who identified as nonbinary:

> It feels very awkward, especially as a nonbinary person, to have . . . my uterus equated to womanhood just entirely. So, I think definitely how hard it is to find unbiased information and to get support that's right for you and just try to make sense of it all. It's just kind of an isolating experience sometimes. (*Riley, early 20s, nonbinary*)

Jaden, another nonbinary individual with PCOS, spoke directly to the woman-centric language used in these online support communities and, additionally, their strong emphasis on fertility, as limiting. Trans and non-binary people feel excluded from conversations about PCOS, explained by Marsh. However, the one exception to this experience in online community support groups seems to be a single Facebook group devoted to individuals with PCOS who identify as queer.

> No one I know in real life actually has it [PCOS] . . . I'm in a couple of Facebook groups. Actually, there's one Facebook group with women—specifically, queer women. Because I found a lot of the focus of the groups outside that are very, very focused on trying to conceive, which is I mean, that's fine, but I don't feel like that's my end goal. And that's not something I feel like I have to do. So, it's very—I'm going to say annoying, but that's not the word I should use— annoying to only have PCOS communities and conversation surrounding trying to conceive and then a lot of the language used is not very inclusive . . . as far as gender and sexuality. So, this queer group that I've frequented is very nice because they don't focus on that. (*Jaden, mid-20s, nonbinary*)

> A lot of information and discussions and pages and things about PCOS and resources . . . are very women-centric . . . it's hard to find information that doesn't just constantly talk about women and women's bodies and women's experiences. . . . I don't want women to not have that, but . . . there's so much that . . . makes trans and nonbinary people feel excluded from being able to talk about their experiences. . . . And, it's hard to . . . constantly be talked over in some of those groups and ignored and sort of shut out and shoved some to the side when the experiences are valid for people like me. (*Marsh, mid-30s, nonbinary*)

Nondisclosure and Social Avoidance

Some of the lack of support described in the prior section may be partially attributable to nondisclosure or social avoidance on the part of the individual living with PCOS. Indeed, these ideas are supported by research on stigmatized identities that has shown less available support may be partially explained by concealment or self-isolation (e.g., Hatzenbuehler et al., 2009). Whereas in general individuals face a dilemma of whether to disclose health-related information (Duggan, 2019), when the information is stigmatizing, the costs of disclosure may be greater. For example, stigma has been linked to social avoidance or decisions not to ask for support in an effort to avoid the feared social rejection if their stigma became known to others (e.g., S. L. Williams et al., 2016). Although to my knowledge, no prior research has examined it, nondisclosure and social avoidance may be a preferred option for some with PCOS, based on narratives describing difficulty talking about PCOS due to shame attached to PCOS symptoms.

Several individuals living with PCOS whom I interviewed, such as Emerson and Jules, spoke of the link between shame attached to symptoms and difficulty talking about them with others:

> Some of the symptoms are hard for people who have PCOS to talk about . . . It can be kind of shameful or embarrassing to talk about having . . . facial hair, body hair, "male pattern" hair loss. . . . All of those things are . . . really hard to deal with and hard to talk about. (*Emerson, mid-30s, nonbinary*)

> People don't know about it [PCOS] or talk about it because . . . it's linked to . . . things that we've been made to feel shameful of, so then we don't talk about it, we brush it under the rug, hushed whispers. . . . People don't want to talk about periods. People don't want to talk about infertility and reproductive issues because we are constantly told that that's something to be ashamed of. (*Jules, late 20s, nonbinary*)

In addition to nondisclosure of PCOS and related symptoms, some with PCOS purposefully avoided specific individuals or social situations. Different symptoms of PCOS, from weight to infertility, were mentioned in relation to social avoidance. Amethyst described the specific challenges of weight and choosing to stay home to avoid being seen by others, whereas Alicia described self-isolating in the context of experiencing miscarriages:

> You don't want to leave the house . . . I'm not comfortable with how this looks and it's not OK to me. . . . It makes me so unmotivated to even try anymore, because I know that it's so hard for me to even shed 5 pounds at this point, especially after having a baby. . . . I had my baby almost a year ago and I still have the baby weight because it just won't go away. . . . It makes me so uncomfortable with myself and I can't find clothes that are comfortable for me to wear. And I don't want to leave the house and so I stay home in pajamas and [do] not leave. (*Amethyst, mid-20s, cisgender woman*)

> After this last one [miscarriage], I have kind of . . . self-isolated, but I'm coming around. But . . . I . . . withdrew from a lot of people after this last miscarriage. I would say that fertility does impact my social relationships . . . I'm a pretty . . . social person, so I like to keep up with people through text, facetime, phone calls and stuff like that. But . . . recently, I haven't been doing any of that. And some people have noticed so I have told them what happened. I guess for me, I don't tell a lot of people . . . right then when it happens, because I don't really

want to be babied during the time. . . . If you're going to give me . . . space to be angry and . . . really express my feelings, fine, but . . . I don't want to be babied, if that makes sense. So that is my reasoning for self-isolating. (*Alicia, early 30s, cisgender woman*)

Although nondisclosure and social avoidance may be directly related to shame surrounding PCOS symptoms, such decisions also may also be tied to their gender diverse and racial/ethnic identities, reflecting additional complexity in navigating social interactions for individuals with PCOS from diverse groups. In what follows, I provide multiple illustrative excerpts from one particular individual with PCOS I interviewed. Farah, a nonbinary individual in their mid-20s, described at multiple points in the interview their nondisclosure and social avoidance. Moreover, their experiences illustrated the interplay of PCOS and gender diverse and racial/ethnic identities in understanding disclosure and avoidance decisions.

Illustrating Farah's Nondisclosure and Purposeful Social Avoidance

From an emotional standpoint . . . there are people I choose not to be around, because I know that they will make comments about how I look. And so . . . one way I cope is just to avoid people that are judgmental towards me, and who I don't feel like I owe an explanation to as to . . . why I have facial hair or . . . why I am the weight I am. And so . . . that's . . . something I do to cope . . . to avoid certain people and surround myself with people who I feel . . . accept me for who I am and who I don't have to . . . give explanations to.

I guess I have talked a little bit about it in therapy, but . . . I have a lot of shame about my symptoms. And so, I really, really don't want to talk about them, even with . . . mental health care providers.

Illustrating Farah's Gender-Specific Issues in Disclosure

It's hard for me, in conversations . . . with other people who have periods who identify as women . . . I have always felt . . . uncomfortable, like I don't have . . . a spot to talk. And I usually just don't, I don't share what my experience is. I just usually . . . pretend . . . I have a regular period, because . . . I know what a period is like, I've had . . . multiple. So . . . I can speak from experience, but I'm not having a period regularly.

Illustrating Ethnic Identity Context in Farah's Nondisclosure and Social Avoidance

Culturally . . . my people are very hairy. And so, for a long time, I just attributed my facial hair to being [racial/ethnic identity] and then finding out that I have PCOS, and that's probably what the cause of it is. And my hair has been an excess amount . . . compared to any of my family members. But . . . I just thought I was kind of an extra hairy [racial/ethnic identity]. . . . we all talk about, a lot, removing our facial hair. And so, it's a little bit more open of a culture . . . with the other women in my [racial/ethnic identity] family in terms of talking about that. And so, people feel like they can make comments about my facial hair. They don't know that I have PCOS. And so, they don't [know] how much it's been a struggle for me (and it's [hair] been a struggle for them, too). And so, I think they have a lot of judgments about it. And so . . . they make comments sometimes. . . . if I go and I haven't just waxed . . . that's kind of uncomfortable for me. And so, . . . at this point in my life, I really avoid seeing my family . . . at all costs, unless I feel a really big obligation. And so . . . I don't always have the greatest relationship with my family because of that, because . . . culturally, we're . . . kind of expected to show up regularly. . . . and that's something I don't do. So, I am often . . . disappointing my family. And, a huge portion of that is due to the fact that . . . they are really judgmental about the way people look. And . . . that's something that I don't want to be around.

Admittedly, individuals I interviewed described a combination of disclosure and nondisclosure of their PCOS, reflecting differences based on individual preferences and individual symptoms. Some individuals, like Ricky, a nonbinary/transmasc individual in their early 40s, described their nondisclosure and desire to keep health status private from others matter-of-factly: "I haven't really disclosed that [PCOS] to a whole lot of people" Others, like Cody, a nonbinary individual in his mid-20s, described being "pretty much an open book" and talking freely about PCOS. Individuals also clarified willingness to disclose particular aspects of PCOS but not others, emphasizing the relative shame attached to hair on particular body parts. Loren, for instance, differentiated a willingness to disclose hairy legs or arms but not hairy nipples. Riley avoided disclosure of certain symptoms in an effort not to draw more attention from others to parts of the body that would increase self-consciousness. Of course, hair removal is another form of nondisclosure or reported in prior research (e.g., Pfister & Rømer, 2017) and in the current narratives, as illustrated by Cynthia.

> I wouldn't tell people that I have . . . hairy nipples. . . . My partners would . . . know that. . . . I wouldn't . . . say that to anybody openly, but would talk about how I have hairy legs or hairy arms. (*Loren, early 20s, nonbinary*)

> If I tell people about it, I—I guess I probably don't go into too much detail about the skin discoloration or mention the skin tags, because obviously if I'm going to mention physical attributes, they're going to . . . notice it more. I don't really want them to do that. So I only mentioned those slightly or not at all. I try not to mention the fact that I tend to sweat a lot because of it. And let's see, I don't go into too much detail about my period, because I guess that can get kind of gross if you actually did. Yeah, so typically things that would encourage people to look at me more intensely or with a sharper eye. I kind of avoid that because I don't want them to focus on the things I'm self-conscious about. (*Riley, early 20s, nonbinary*)

I mean, being hairy is something I try to hide. And it's not something I'm terribly comfortable discussing with a lot of people, that I have to take extra effort to remove hair all over. (*Cynthia, mid-30s, cisgender woman*)

Quite by contrast to the many reports of nondisclosure or self-isolating due to symptoms of PCOS, many also described *purposeful* disclosure of PCOS. It appeared that in these cases disclosure was a means of coping and a way to call much-needed attention to the condition. As mentioned in the following two excerpts, individuals with PCOS also disclosed as a way to help others who might be struggling with similar PCOS symptoms. Future research should examine the extent of such purposeful disclosure in PCOS.

Well, I'm . . . totally an open-book type of person, so if someone asks me, I'm actually really passionate about . . . letting other women know . . . I feel like a lot of women don't know about their own menstrual health, and that's a huge issue. So if I talk about it, maybe . . . some people will be like, "huh, maybe something's wrong with me" or "I'll go get checked out.". . . So I tell a lot of people. (*Jackie, early 20s, cisgender woman*)

Anything that I deal with, I try to bring awareness to because I don't want someone to . . . think that they're the only person going through it. And if I can help anyone, that's what I'm here for. . . . I feel as though women of color are more likely to . . . go through something like this alone rather than sharing their experience. I don't know if it's . . . an embarrassment thing, but it's just something I've made note of. (*Alicia, early 30s, cisgender woman*)

Pressure to Conform to Femininity: Social Control in Close Relationships

Some of the lacking social support and intentional social avoidance appeared to stem from behaviors of others, reflecting the possibility that individuals with PCOS might not feel supported by others from whom support is available. In particular, this section considers the pressures individuals with PCOS encounter from close others to change their bodies in ways that conform to expectations for females. Many individuals, such as Cody and Jules, described pressures to conform from their family—especially their mothers—and particularly around body hair. Jules described feelings of humiliation after receiving hair removal equipment from their mother, who gifted it as a means of helping them fit in with cultural expectations of hairlessness:

Facial hair is something that she [my mom] didn't want for me . . . she was raised to see . . . somebody with facial hair as outside the norm and . . . they should conform and fit in. . . . So I think there was always a push . . . from my mom for me to be . . . feminine and to fit in with society . . . as a woman. (*Cody, mid-20s, nonbinary*)

I remember my mother for Christmas when . . . I was . . . a kid, I would be sitting there under the tree and I would unwrap . . . facial hair shaving devices.

And then when I was completely crestfallen and—and humiliated . . . thanks for reminding me that I have facial hair that's disgusting, Mom. . . . I would then be reprimanded for not being grateful because, well, they're just trying to help you. (*Jules, late 20s, nonbinary*)

Whereas this or similar behaviors from family members are meant to "help" individuals with PCOS to avoid social rejection from the outside world, the "helpful" behaviors themselves are experienced as socially rejecting. In concept, pressure to conform to femininity or other expectations from close others may share some similarity with health-related social control efforts from the literature on close relationships. With health-related social control, close others persuade their loved ones to engage in healthy behaviors or deter them from unhealthy ones (Umberson, 1987). For example, close others may encourage individuals toward positive behavior change, such as exercise or eating patterns (e.g., Lewis & Rook, 1999). Some evidence suggests social control can be effective in bringing about health behavior change; however, the choice of strategy matters. Whereas positive control attempts, such as positive reinforcement and using logic or modeling of the healthy behavior, can be effective at bringing out healthy behaviors or deterring unhealthy ones, negative control attempts, such as making a loved one feel bad about themselves or their health, are not (Lewis & Butterfield, 2005).

It may be that the social control efforts of family members of individuals living with PCOS would be classified as the negative type of control attempts, at least by the recipient with PCOS. Even if positive intentions underlie these social control efforts, in the context of weight or other characteristics that are stigmatized (like PCOS symptoms), they may be interpreted as stigma rather than positive attempts to help with health improvement. Taking the common symptom of PCOS of obesity for example, weight-based social control in particular often backfires and leads to worse health behaviors (e.g., Brunson et al., 2014). A recent study of more than 600 young women found that positive social control behaviors (e.g., praise, using positive emotion) from mothers predicted more healthy eating, physical activity, and body appreciation, whereas negative social control behaviors (e.g., guilt, using negative emotion) predicted less healthy eating, physical activity, and body appreciation and more body dissatisfaction (Arroyo et al., 2020). Individuals classified as overweight and obese in general have self-reported that their worst experiences with weight stigma most often originated from family— even if attempts to motivate weight loss come from genuine concern for one's health (Puhl et al., 2008). Although no studies have specifically looked at social control attempts by loved ones in PCOS, parents of individuals with

PCOS are a source of distress when making comments about weight (Weiss & Bulmer, 2011).

In my own case of being obese and living with PCOS, I was the recipient of multiple attempts by family members to encourage weight loss in my teens and early 20s. These attempts would be classified as the negative type of social control because they involved fear and shaming tactics. In one particular example, my mother wrote me a letter in which she described her concern for my future and my ability to find a husband because no boys wanted to date fat girls. She pleaded with me to lose weight. Of course, because of the lack of understanding of PCOS, she had not considered that PCOS could be causing my weight gain or contributing to my inability to lose weight.

Some individuals living with PCOS that I interviewed described their attempts to navigate the world in which loved ones judged their weight, as described earlier. Dylan, for example, poignantly described maintaining the illusion of being a "good fatty" in front of close others to avoid the social consequences, while satisfying real hunger in private with food choices that would have been deemed unhealthy in the eyes of onlooking others:

> There's a secretive layer to my life. Like I think I learned when I was in fourth grade that . . . I would get chastised by my parents for . . . wanting seconds, which resulted in like, waiting for everyone to go to bed and then raiding the refrigerator. And so there became like this hidden layer of like what people see me eat and like what I devoured in private . . . in college, for example, I would go to fast food, eat really fast in my car and . . . hide the trash before anyone saw . . . part of me was hidden because of the social pressure to . . . navigate food in a particular way and be seen as a "good fatty" . . . there's a lot of health moralism . . . and . . . I need to perform in a way that is . . . a "good fatty" . . . I . . . eat the healthy things . . . just demonstrate behaviors that . . . people perceive as healthy. (*Dylan, late 20s, genderqueer*)

Instead of social control efforts from others being helpful, pressure from others to conform may be more akin to microaggressions, or those everyday slights or comments people say that unintentionally offend the individual with the stigmatized condition or identity. Often, we think of microaggressions as experienced by minoritized racial/ethnic groups or other marginalized groups in society. They might also apply to those who are overweight, particularly when people think they are well intentioned or want to help others fit in; meanwhile, these efforts are experienced as judgmental and rejecting. Moreover, how "good" these intentions are in the context of weight is questionable given that people actually believe that their blatantly demeaning remarks about others' weight are justified for the good of the obese person (Major et al., 2012). To my knowledge, no research has yet examined the experience of social control efforts or microaggressions in PCOS.

Finally, cultural context may undergird or even exacerbate these pressures to conform or familial efforts of social control. That is, pressures to conform to feminine standards may originate in one's racial/ethnic identity such that it becomes an element of their culture. Jules's narrative pointed to strong cultural views on femininity as source of these pressures from families:

> One of my biggest and most prominent symptoms has been body and facial hair. And because that's still externally visible . . . it's been . . . a constant . . . issue . . . I remember growing up . . . I started to get . . . sideburns . . . and it got to the point where my mother, every single time I would leave the house from when I was young to when I left the house as . . . a late teenager, she would always be like, "be careful to hide your sideburns" or "aren't you going to shave?" . . . I was constantly being told to fix this, fix that . . . shave this, shave that. . . . I do think I was affected culturally by my mother because she came from a very binary culture . . . she would constantly criticize me for my femininity or lack thereof. (*Jules, late 20s, nonbinary*)

Admittedly, standards for women's bodies for some racial or ethnic identities may allow for greater flexibility, such as greater allowance for higher body weight or body hair. Yet those I interviewed directly addressed this issue, clarifying that, despite any greater flexibility, there still is a "line" that people of color should not cross to meet expectations. In an illustrative example from an individual of color I interviewed, Riley described these culturally based pressures:

> I've been . . . really hairy all my life. . . . I . . . chalked it up to just being a woman of color. . . . But . . . growing up, it definitely made me feel . . . really bad and really othered . . . even among my own people, I still felt very much like an outsider. . . . There's so much pressure to . . . be completely hairless when you leave your house. So that was a big stressor for me all the time growing up and through high school and even now, college as well. . . . if you're even at all coded as a woman, people expect you to perform really high feminine standards . . . so if you're somebody who is fat or has a lot of . . . acne or facial hair or body hair that's hard to keep down because it's exhausting to have to shave and tweeze every day, they judge you a lot. Because you're not performing to those standards. . . . It's exhausting to have to do that and obviously I can't really control what I look like or what my body does, with the exception of using medication for it. . . . I have received a lot of judgment . . . sometimes . . . well-intentioned, concerned comments, but . . . things that were . . . ultimately unhelpful or even hurtful because it's not like I could do anything about it. . . . it has really impacted how I saw myself and how I was treated even back where I lived in [home country], where because we're people of color, more people expect them to be curvier and hairier. But . . . there's still this line . . . you can't be past. . . . This is an acceptable level of difference, but you can't cross that line or else you're just unsightly or somehow not conforming well enough. (*Riley, early 20s, nonbinary*)

Support From Like Others and Positive Social Experiences

Despite a clear need for more PCOS-specific support, many individuals with PCOS spoke of the positive impact that PCOS has had on their social relationships. In particular, support from others who also were diagnosed with PCOS frequently presented in these positive social encounters. This experience is illustrated by Alia, who described how support from similar others can make one feel understood, which is important when experiencing a condition that can impact every aspect of life. Indeed, prior published work has found online PCOS support helpful particularly because friends and family do not understand the experience (Ee et al., 2020; S. Williams et al., 2015). Perhaps, too, it is helpful because PCOS is such an invisible condition, and relating with similar others seemed especially validating for individuals living with PCOS.

> There has been a positivity coming out of it [PCOS], in that I'm a member of several PCOS groups on social media. And these people are very supportive. They're supportive of many different types of people who have PCOS. They're very uplifting. And I feel like I've found some really, truly caring people who have PCOS who are trying their best to reach out to other people. Because as I said before, we all kind of feel lost. So, it's . . . very helpful to just be a member of one of these groups, even if you don't post, just to see that there's other people asking questions that you might want to ask. And the group . . . or the community is strong. . . . I think when you have a body condition, it is so deeply ingrained inside of you that it affects basically everything, and it's so important to have other people who at least somewhat understand you. And, so, I've seen something very beautiful come out of that. (*Alia, early 30s, cisgender woman*)

Support from others with PCOS may be especially helpful in the context of particular symptoms with which individuals are struggling. For example, Alicia shared that after her miscarriages, connecting on social media with others going through infertility was part of her coping process:

> As far as my fertility journey, journaling helps me a lot. Getting . . . keepsakes or jewelry . . . to represent the angel babies . . . helps me too. I've gotten tattoos. Ink therapy is therapy for me. . . . and honestly, reading the experiences of others helps me. . . . I follow a lot of . . . Instagram accounts where people are . . . discussing their fertility . . . journey, most of them a lot different from mine because I guess my issue is not getting pregnant, it's staying pregnant, but I still like seeing the happy endings for other people and seeing how they get to the other side. (*Alicia, early 30s, cisgender woman*)

However, talking about PCOS with friends and family, whether or not they themselves had PCOS, appeared to strengthen the bonds of the relationships. Social benefits might be garnered from disclosing PCOS diagnosis and struggles more generally, not just with similar others with PCOS. One published qualitative study of adolescent girls with PCOS in England found similarly strengthened relationships after sharing PCOS diagnosis with friends and family (G. L. Jones et al., 2011). Two excerpts by Deidre illustrate this strengthening in the context of close friendships as well as family member relationships:

> Having . . . that network of friends that I could talk to about it was really good. I feel like that really strengthened our relationship, that we were able to talk about this issue and . . . then it . . . opened up to . . . things . . . they've gone through. . . . One of my friends told me about her thyroid disorder, and we . . . bonded over the fact that we were both going to endocrinologists. So, I feel like in that respect it was really good. (*Deidre, mid-20s, cisgender woman*)

> I've talked to quite a few of my family members about it. My sister especially . . . I . . . never knew that she had gone through similar things as me . . . having . . . irregular periods and . . . I knew she had acne. . . . And . . . she really wants to have kids in the future. And . . . knowing that she might struggle to have kids because of PCOS . . . broke my heart a little bit, but I feel like that made our relationship stronger . . . being able to talk about PCOS and how it might affect each other and . . . knowing that when she tries to have kids, she'll have me there who . . . understands . . . what PCOS is about. (*Deidre, mid-20s, cisgender woman*)

More unexpectedly, individuals living with PCOS garnered additional support from others who were experiencing challenges other than PCOS. A source of support in individuals with PCOS whom I interviewed was individuals with diverse sex and gender identities. Regardless of their own gender, some individuals I interviewed found the more flexible gender expectations surrounding nonbinary or transgender identities helpful for their own reframing of their gender-violating PCOS symptoms, such as body hair. This support from different others occurred mostly online, which fits with prior research in the area of online community support (Wright et al., 2020). The online environment of social media, such as Instagram and Facebook, presumably allows for greater access to diverse groups and their experiences. One illustrative example is an excerpt by Marsh, who described feeling validated by the experiences of intersex individuals:

> So, I think obviously my situation is pretty different than a lot of people who have PCOS who identify as women . . . I feel like it mostly is a positive thing for me in making me feel sort of secure about my gender identity. . . . I've been a lesbian . . . and now I'm . . . perceived as a gay man. I am bi, I am trans, and I'm intersex. . . . I saw a couple of speakers who are intersex and, obviously in different ways than I am because they were people who are . . . androgen insensitive . . . and had . . . undescended testes . . . and had surgeries performed on them. And I don't want to say that I totally understand the experience of that,

but I feel sort of validated by having talked to them about my experiences . . . this has helped me to . . . be closer to people and not hold this shame about . . . my body hair, my health, as if it's something that I had control of. So, opening up about it has been really good for me and for being vulnerable and close to people. (*Marsh, mid-30s, nonbinary*)

Jean's narrative discussed support gained by following the social media site of a nonbinary individual with PCOS. Even though Jean did not identify as nonbinary, the body positivity and normalizing of body hair of the nonbinary individual felt supportive to her:

I feel like I end up seeking out not necessarily support, but . . . things that make me feel solidarity from outside of PCOS spaces. . . . I follow this person on Instagram who is a nonbinary person who wears—has a very feminine aesthetic and also has a lot of hair on their body, and so they post a lot about . . . navigating the judgment that they receive from the world and coming to a space of accepting their body just as it is and not feeling . . . they have to shave because that's what the world wants them to do, not feeling like it limits their ability to tap into their femininity. But really just stand firm in their gender identity. And so . . . I get . . . some sense of . . . "your body is OK" . . . but it's also . . . still not perfect, because I'm not nonbinary . . . I need there to be more . . . spaces where it's . . . OK to be a woman who has excess hair. It's OK to have—to hold on to that gender identity and not conform to these standards . . . the amount of hair that you have on your body does not define what your gender identity is. And we need to be able to say, that's OK if you're nonbinary, that's OK if you're a woman, that's OK if you're a man. (*Jean, late 20s, cisgender woman*)

In sum, this first half of the chapter described ways that individuals experienced social support, or lack thereof, and related processes in the context of PCOS. Despite the fact that some individuals reported positive relationship impacts of PCOS through bringing them closer to their networks and being helped by contact with similar others, many perceived PCOS support to be unavailable. These findings, along with the limited prior research, underscore the importance of future research and advocacy work that considers the unique close relationship and especially support needs of diverse groups living with PCOS.

SEXUALITY, PARTNER RELATIONS, AND DATING IN PCOS

In this second part of the chapter, I explore the impact of PCOS on sexuality and more intimate relationships (partners, dating). Like with social support, PCOS may be associated with both negative and positive elements of sexuality and relationships, which may further vary by gender self-identification.

Sexual Functioning and Body Image in PCOS

Does PCOS have an impact on sexual functioning? Given the lack of PCOS research in many areas of psychosocial functioning, I was pleased to find at least a small body of existing research on sexual functioning in individuals with PCOS. I briefly review that literature here before describing the experiences reported by individuals I interviewed. Overall, my takeaway is that published findings on sexual functioning are mixed but with mostly weak evidence for worse sexual functioning in PCOS. Although some studies find sexual dissatisfaction in reports of those with PCOS (Amiri et al., 2014), others find no differences in sexual functioning when comparing individuals with and without PCOS (e.g., Morotti et al., 2013). When comparing individuals with untreated PCOS to control participants, at least one study found worse sexual functioning in only one area (less orgasm/completion than controls) with similarities in the other areas (similar levels of pleasure/satisfaction, desire/frequency, desire/interest, and arousal/excitement; Stovall et al., 2012). This similarity in sexual functioning between those with and without PCOS is further supported by a recent systematic review and meta-analysis that synthesized data from 2,626 participants across 10 studies, finding no association between PCOS and female sexual dysfunction (Zhao et al., 2019).

Still, it may be that specific PCOS symptoms such as body size and body hair create problems for sexual functioning that are not captured when researchers make general comparisons between those with and without PCOS (Eftekhar et al., 2014; Zhao et al., 2019). In fact, there is accumulating evidence that body weight and shape associated with PCOS may contribute to less sexual satisfaction or worsened functioning. Here is the gist of these findings that support this idea. First, when comparing sexual functioning in groups classified as normal weight individuals with and without PCOS, research has found no difference in sexual functioning, indicating PCOS diagnosis alone does not contribute to sexual functioning (Morotti et al., 2013). Second, when comparing sexual functioning (desire, sexual excitement, orgasm, satisfaction) in individuals classified as obese with and without PCOS, research finds similar sexuality-related outcomes (Zueff et al., 2015), again indicating that PCOS diagnosis alone does not contribute to sexual functioning but perhaps weight might. Third, that same study (Zueff et al., 2015) showed lower scores on sexuality-related outcomes based on waist-to-hip ratio indicative of less feminine presentation of body shape contributing to sexual functioning rather than PCOS diagnosis per se. Fourth, and finally, another study found less orgasm/completion (one indicator of sexual functioning/satisfaction) in individuals with PCOS, especially when they had higher body mass index (BMI) scores (Stovall et al., 2012). Taken together, these findings may imply that PCOS diagnosis itself may not link with worse sexual outcomes but rather that body shape and weight may be the primary factors.

If body shape and weight do influence sexual functioning in PCOS, body image may be how they manifest their impact. Attitudes that individuals hold about their bodies can explain different levels of sexual satisfaction (Chrisler & Johnston-Robledo, 2018). Indeed, a review of 57 studies showed that body image can affect all aspects of female sexual functioning (Woertman & van den Brink, 2012). For example, negative body image can lead to self-consciousness or mental distraction during sex, which interferes with sexual arousal (Wiederman, 2001). Aligned with this possibility, some studies have found correlations between negative body image and poorer sexual functioning in PCOS. A study of individuals with PCOS in Brazil whose BMI scores ranged from normal to obese found that body dissatisfaction was uniquely related to worse sexual functioning (Kogure et al., 2019). In a German study, researchers found that women with PCOS ($n = 50$) were less satisfied with their sexual lives and perceived themselves as less attractive than age-matched women without PCOS ($n = 50$; Elsenbruch et al., 2003). Further, those with PCOS also perceived that their partners were less satisfied with their sexual lives and found them less attractive.

Those with PCOS I interviewed also commonly revealed a connection between negative body image and sexuality, regardless of gender identity. As illustrated in the excerpts that follow, Josie, Angelina, and Farah spoke to this connection.

> I don't like being intimate with other people for the most part . . . I don't really have sex for the most part, because I'm afraid of other people seeing my body. (*Josie, early 20s, cisgender woman*)

> The weight can sometimes make me feel less desirable. Although, my husband has never made me feel that way. (*Angelina, late 30s, cisgender woman*)

> I have a lot of anxieties around having sex, because I have such a negative body image. Sometimes I avoid having sex, because I feel bad about how I look. (*Farah, mid-20s, nonbinary*)

Although less frequently discussed, PCOS may affect sexual outcomes because of menstrual and pelvic pain that limits one's physical ability to have sex, which supports Zhao and colleagues' (2019) mention of direct and indirect factors that might contribute to sexual functioning. During her interview, Alia described how pain during intimacy or even depression related to PCOS creates challenges to sexual relationships with partners. Vaginal dryness, perceived to be related to PCOS, may also have a direct impact on sexual functioning, as illustrated by Kendall's excerpt.

> I am a sexual person and I do have a husband. We are intimate with each other and we seem to have a good sex life. But the pain issue has affected me. . . . I've had severe pain during intimacy . . . such that I've had to stop . . . also, when I'm very depressed . . . there's no way I can be as intimate with my husband. So really, it does affect me. But the good thing is . . . I have a very understanding husband, who has known me for so long. He's seen me gain all that weight, and he's seen me lose it. Let's put it like that. . . . He's really seen it, so he understands I really have a problem. So, he's always been very supportive and understanding. (*Alia, early 30s, cisgender woman*)

> The vaginal dryness that I experience is very self-esteem lowering as well when it comes to having an intimate relationship with my partner and not feeling embarrassed about my condition. (*Kendall, early 20s, nonbinary*)

Exploring Positive Sexuality in PCOS

Importantly, the negative impact of PCOS-related body image on sexuality was not present for all. To my knowledge, no prior research has uncovered positive elements to sexual relationships in the context of PCOS. Narratives here suggest that positive sexuality in the context of PCOS may partly depend on partner preferences that are directly related to gender and sexual orientation. For example, some individuals with gender diverse identities experienced positive elements of sexuality because of more flexible appearance-related expectations within the queer community. As illustrated in the following excerpt, Jo described the benefit of being queer as not having to perform femininity for straight men. Simultaneously, however, they still experienced challenges related to PCOS-related body hair when queer partners were not attracted to masculine characteristics. Cody described challenges encountered with cisgender men as well, and how he now chooses queer partners.

> I've always identified as queer to some level. And, I think that's, in some ways, been a blessing, because I never felt like I had to look a certain way or perform a certain way to be enough for a straight man. So, that's . . . taken [away] some of the burden that many straight ciswomen with PCOS feel. . . . I've had some challenges with my current partner, who's a lesbian . . . she supports me doing what feels good for me but has also told me that . . . the amount of body hair I have is not attractive to her. It feels too masculine and she doesn't want to be with . . . a man or somebody who's like a man. (*Jo, late 20s, genderqueer/ nonbinary*)

> I've always identified as . . . bisexual or pansexual, but I've always had a lot of trouble with cis men and my body hair. And it's been hard to . . . explain . . .

why I'm not doing anything about it. Because people don't tend to understand why you don't want to fit into their boxes. . . . I haven't had trouble with . . . queer people I've dated. Queer people just see you as you are and . . . take you for what you are. . . . But . . . with cis men, . . . they make such a big stink over the smallest little things because most of the ones that I've experienced, . . . expect you to conform. So, it's been a little frustrating dating certain types of people. But I've mostly surrounded myself with queer people and queer friends and queer relationships. So, it hasn't been—it hasn't been so bad recently. (*Cody, mid-20s, nonbinary*)

Positive sexuality was also reported for other reasons across gender identity. Some reported sexual relations as positively influenced by irregular menstruation due to PCOS. Rory, for example, described not having to worry about being on a period to have sex (although they also described missing the opportunity for having sex while menstruating; i.e., "period sex"):

The biggest thing with PCOS is . . . not having a regular period. And so that means that I can have . . . period-free sex a lot more than people who have periods, so I don't have to think about it as much. But . . . on the flip side, . . . I've had period sex, and I enjoyed that. But I don't know when my period's coming. So, I can't really . . . plan and look forward to it, or . . . plan around it, but also . . . less of that. So, there's good and bad. (*Rory, early 20s, nonbinary*)

Others reported an increased libido that they attributed to PCOS and experienced as positive in their lives. One example from the interviews is Leah, who described an intense libido and using masculinizing symptoms of PCOS in positive ways, such as embracing it in sexual scenarios:

I feel like it [PCOS] makes my body look more masculine. . . . My belly is bigger than my breasts . . . and I don't have very big hips. . . . I . . . wish I had . . . more of a pear than an apple shape, but . . . you get what you get. Sometimes I really use that masculinity in ways that I really enjoyed. Like when I let myself go to a more masculine place, . . . sometimes I'm more masculine in bed with people. . . . Usually I . . . can roll with that. (*Leah, mid-40s, cisgender(ish) woman*)

Some talked about the possibility that increased testosterone in their bodies contributed to increased libido, as evidenced by Jack's conversation with a physician.

PCOS has impacted my sexuality . . . one of the things that I have had mixed experiences with, that sometimes it's been a positive, sometimes it's been a negative, is . . . I've always had a much more intense libido than my partners. And I remember talking to my doctor about this, too, and saying . . . does my PCOS impact this at all? Because I have different hormone levels than other people. And she said, yes, probably. (*Jack, mid-30s, nonbinary*)

However, the science linking hormones and increased libido in those with PCOS seems equivocal. More research is needed to distinguish when or for whom androgens such as testosterone contribute to hirsutism and therefore negative body image and poorer sexual outcomes versus increased sexual desire (Zhao et al., 2019). One recent study found increased sexual desire and masturbation frequency associated with more severe PCOS symptoms (e.g., hirsutism), suggesting links between androgens and desire; however, desire may not equate to increased sexual behavior (Tzalazidis & Oinonen, 2021). The limited scientific understanding appears to trickle down into the lived experiences of those with PCOS, as evidenced by some I interviewed who were uncertain whether PCOS was the cause of their libido. As the focus of this chapter is not on the biological underpinnings of PCOS experience, I will not offer further discussion of the potential role of increased androgens with PCOS sexuality.

In conclusion, more psychological research is needed on the sexual lives (not just the sexual functioning) of individuals living with PCOS. At this point, it is unclear in the scientific literature whether sexual experiences are linked to PCOS (directly or indirectly). The vast majority of published research that does exist on the sexual lives of those with PCOS has focused on sexual functioning, which may point to a negative impact of body size and shape, and therefore body image, relating to sexual satisfaction. Additionally, no studies have intentionally examined the positive sexual experiences or pleasure experienced by individuals living with PCOS. In fact, Leah highlighted the possibility of specific sexual pleasure possible *because of* living in a larger body attributable to PCOS.

> Maybe . . . there's this . . . powerful, juicy sexuality to bigger women and to bigger women with PCOS, and we don't talk about that part. We talk about . . . they're fat and it's terrible. We don't talk about . . . pleasure and access to pleasure and what . . . all this extra testosterone does. . . . And I can't believe that there's nothing there. (*Leah, mid-40s, cisgender(ish) woman*)

Partner Relationships and Dating

Given the overall lack of research on PCOS, you may not be surprised to learn that I could not locate published studies on how PCOS impacts relationships with partners or dating. However, it was clear in the narratives of individuals I interviewed that living with PCOS does have an impact on aspects of relationships and dating beyond assessments of sexual functioning, which has been the focus of prior research on intimate relationships. For example, issues regarding sexuality and body image that individuals attributed to PCOS had some impact on their close relationship partners. Jack, for example, struggled with more intense sexual desire and negotiating that intensity with sexual partners:

> I've always struggled with the fact that I've had a much more . . . intense sexual desire than other people that I've been with in my life. And that's . . . always just been a weird experience for me . . . that's not something that I've ever talked to other people with PCOS about, now that I think about it out loud. Part of me kind of wishes that I—I had. I'm sure my experience is not universal by any means, because I know for some people, sex is complicated because they're dealing with chronic pain all the time. . . . I wish that that would be something that . . . could come up in spaces more . . . it's been a personal struggle of mine to help partners I've had to understand where I'm coming from without seeming like I'm just . . . insatiable or something. . . . because it's never been about pressuring. It's just more like when I've talked to people, [they] just don't get [my] experience. (*Jack, mid-30s, nonbinary*)

By contrast, Cynthia described body image issues related to weight gain resulting from PCOS as problematic for her sexual desire in her relationship with her husband. She described him as supportive and communicative, but she worried about the impact of her body image and sexual functioning on him.

> I think lately it's been more of a negative impact on our sexual relationship and probably because I've been really in my head over gaining weight. But I will say, my husband is very supportive, and we've been very good at communicating very openly about it. And, that's very helpful, because I don't want him to feel rejected, so . . . having a conversation like, look, I'm feeling gross right now. It's nothing personal. (*Cynthia, mid-30s, cisgender woman*)

Similar concerns related to weight and body image issues in PCOS influenced dating lives for those not yet partnered. Some individuals I interviewed described avoiding dating entirely due to negative body image and body consciousness brought about by specific symptoms of PCOS. Tina and Megan both described how their weight made them not want to date in general or until after weight loss, and Jean described the impact of excess body hair on dating.

> Yeah, for me, it really does go to the weight gain. I don't think that you have to be thin to date, but because of my own hang-ups, my body makes me not want to date. (*Tina, late 20s, cisgender woman*)

> I've never actually dated anyone. I've never been in a relationship with anyone before. . . . I always think "I need to lose weight before I can actually meet someone" or "I need to lose weight to even be noticed by people." I think that's a big factor. (*Megan, early 20s, cisgender woman*)

> I have a lot of anxiety about what people will think about my body. So I tend not to let people get too close or not really commit to pursuing relationships romantically, because . . . if I'm . . . hitting it off with someone and things are going great . . . I have this thought in the back of my head . . . "What if this keeps going and what if they want to hook up . . . what am I going to do about my body . . . what am I going to do about all this hair on my body?" . . . And then . . . instead of . . . being like . . . let's see what happens . . . I'm like, let me shut this down right now so I don't ever have to get to that bridge. (*Jean, late 20s, cisgender woman*)

Others worried that dating would not even be an option for them because of their appearance, which they attributed to PCOS. Jules described being told their entire life they were unattractive and internalized that message such that dating did not even seem a possibility. Similarly, Amy believed dating would not be possible because of others' negative judgments about her appearance. She worried that due to masculinizing features of PCOS, potential dating partners would erroneously perceive her as gender diverse or a lesbian on online dating apps.

> I had such low self-confidence and feeling very unattractive because I'd basically been told my entire life that I didn't fit what was considered attractive nor what fit as woman. So why would I even be considered? . . . which, again, horrible mentality, but these are the things that had been said to me. . . . And so, basically, for me, . . . relationships didn't even enter into my head, because why would they? . . . Even if I wanted to, . . . there were no people that would have crushes on me. (*Jules, late 20s, nonbinary*)

> If I'm on . . . a dating app . . . people might see my picture and just . . . skip over my name and just assume that . . . I'm either . . . a guy . . . like, I'm trans and I just haven't changed my name or that I'm just like a full blown stereotypical . . . butch lesbian, which is also not the case. (*Amy, mid-20s, cisgender woman*)

Amy and others went on to describe what reflected a darker side or negative implication of the body image and confidence issues brought about by PCOS symptoms. Amy worried of being at risk for attracting less than desirable partners:

> As far as . . . the overweight thing goes, trying to . . . find people to go on dates with can be tough sometimes, especially . . . with . . . dating apps and things like that. People can be cruel, sometimes without even realizing . . . it makes it harder for people to kind of take you seriously or it might attract . . . some people that you don't necessarily want to get involved with. (*Amy, mid-20s, cisgender woman*)

This concern was supported by others who described risky sexual behaviors or abuse in relationships they felt resulted from confidence or body image issues. Jules, for instance, connected their low self-confidence related to PCOS to an entanglement in an abusive relationship:

At 18–19, I wound up getting into an abusive relationship for 5 years . . . I'm not blaming everything on PCOS, of course, . . . but . . . my low self-confidence, the fact that I didn't feel feminine enough . . . when somebody did then show interest in me, while being a toxic individual who even in the relationship would give me issues for my body hair and stuff like that . . . had I had any confidence in myself . . . had I not basically been in an emotionally already wrecked and vulnerable state, I probably would not have jumped into the first relationship with the first man that showed interest in me. (*Jules, late 20s, nonbinary*)

These narratives suggest that individuals with PCOS who are encountering body image issues may not date or may feel forced to choose unhealthy relationships because of their personal histories of not being attractive to other potential dating partners. Additionally, although reported less frequently, individuals may find dating a challenge due to the potential for future infertility problems. As Josie described, she avoided dating because she had negative reactions from prior partners after disclosing information about her potential for infertility:

I don't ever want to get too close to someone because . . . I don't want them to be scared away by my illness or have it be too much for them to handle. And then I just get my feelings hurt. So, I tend not to date. And if I do date, it's very rare. It takes me a long time to trust someone and let them in. . . . A lot of guys don't want to date a girl with reproductive issues because they want kids when they're older. That's . . . a hard part about dating . . . if they really want kids when we're married and I can't give them kids. . . . for the most part, I date for marriage. So that's why dating is especially hard with PCOS, because a lot of the guys I dated in the past have wanted kids. And then when I told them I can't have kids or it will be very hard when I'm older to have kids, they see that as drama or complications that they don't want in their life. So. They usually break up with me. (*Josie, early 20s, cisgender woman*)

As this chapter is the first to report some of these findings reflecting what I would describe as a web of linkages among body image, identity, sexuality, and dating in PCOS, future research should explore in more depth the intimate and sexual relations in individuals living with PCOS.

CONCLUSION

This chapter described the close relationship processes reported by individuals living with PCOS whom I interviewed. Although prior research literature has examined the sexual functioning in the lives of individuals with PCOS, even that work is limited in size and scope. Narratives from those I interviewed revealed several impacts of PCOS on close relationship processes, many of which were never before examined in research and therefore need further exploration. These include pressures or social control attempts from close others to change their bodies to conform to societal standards for femininity, lack of social support, positive support from both similar (those with PCOS) and dissimilar (diverse sex and genders) others, and challenges with sexuality and dating due to body image. Again, glaringly absent from any PCOS research is attention to diverse gender identity in relationship processes of individuals living with PCOS. In the next chapter, I explore the psychological risks attached to PCOS and its symptoms and, quite by contrast, the potential for psychological growth.

5 PSYCHOLOGICAL RISK AND GROWTH IN PCOS

Those of us who stand outside the circle of this society's definition of acceptable women; those of us who have been forged in the crucibles of difference— those of us who are poor, who are lesbians, who are Black, who are older— know that survival is not an academic skill. . . . *It is learning how to take our differences and make them strengths.*

–Audre Lorde (1984, p. 112), *Sister Outsider*

This fifth chapter of the book explores whether and how PCOS impacts psychological outcomes. In this chapter, I review the evidence that individuals living with polycystic ovary syndrome (PCOS) are at increased risk for psychological outcomes of depression, anxiety, and worse quality of life (QOL) and the potential reasons why, offering excerpts from individuals living with PCOS that I interviewed to further illustrate the reasons. These risks, along with their explanations, speak to areas of vulnerability in the lives of individuals living with PCOS that interventions could target to improve psychological outcomes. However, and importantly, individuals I interviewed also reported psychological growth stemming from PCOS, suggesting that less

https://doi.org/10.1037/0000337-006
The Psychology of PCOS: Building the Science and Breaking the Silence, by S. L. Williams

negative or more positive outcomes are already possible. Given that psychological growth in the face of PCOS has not been discussed previously, this chapter breaks new ground in research on psychological outcomes in PCOS.

PCOS AND PSYCHOLOGICAL RISK

In examining the scientific literature for what we know so far about psychological risks in PCOS, I was surprised to find a relatively expansive literature. Indeed, when researching most other psychosocial aspects of PCOS discussed in this book, I found rather limited literatures. This work on psychological risk in PCOS, however, mostly comes out of medical rather than psychological science. Even still, in the medical literature, PCOS research on psychological outcomes represents a small percentage of the total (Himelein & Thatcher, 2006b). This is despite that the total amount of PCOS-related citations increased at least fivefold in the 15 years since 2006.

Although research on psychological disorders in the general population shows high rates of co-occurring anxiety and depression (Kessler et al., 2005), those with PCOS are at even greater risk for these negative psychological outcomes, compared with their counterparts without PCOS (Dokras et al., 2011, 2012). Some suggest that other psychological disorders may also be increased in those with PCOS (eating disorders, bipolar disorder, attention-deficit/hyperactivity disorder; Rodriguez-Paris et al., 2019), but this work is currently much more limited in scope. As such, I focus this chapter on evidence of depression, anxiety, as well as QOL. Moreover, because of the large number of individual studies on the psychological outcomes of depression, anxiety, and QOL, I mainly describe results of review papers or meta-analyses, which capture overarching takeaway messages because they summarize data from multiple studies at once. The strength in the meta-analytic technique lies in the combining of data across multiple studies rather than just one. Of course, not even this robust technique can counteract the limitations related to study design (cross-sectional rather than longitudinal) and samples (lacking diversity) that I outlined in Chapter 1.

Increased Risk for Anxiety and Depression and Lower Quality of Life in PCOS

Let us now consider the evidence for the increased risk of depression, anxiety, and (later) lower QOL in individuals living with PCOS. Probably the best evidence we currently have are the two meta-analyses published in 2011 and 2012, which separately examined risk for anxiety and depression in those with PCOS. After combining the results of four cross-sectional studies that compared patients with PCOS and control individuals without PCOS, meta-analytic results revealed that prevalence of anxiety was higher in individuals living with PCOS; indeed, they were 6 to nearly 7 times more likely to have anxiety symptoms compared with counterparts without PCOS (Dokras et al., 2012). Similarly, after combining results of 10 cross-sectional studies of depression, meta-analytic results revealed those with PCOS were 4 times more likely to have abnormal scores indicative of depression compared with individuals without PCOS (Dokras et al., 2011). This finding remained after considering the body mass index (BMI, a ratio of weight [kilograms] divided by height [square meters]) of those with PCOS (i.e., studies either used BMI-matched control individuals or found no difference in BMI between PCOS and non-PCOS groups). Although studies do not specify that PCOS caused depression and anxiety, some have found newly diagnosed disorders follow rather than precede PCOS diagnosis (Hung et al., 2014).

To clarify further the severity of these psychological risks in PCOS, let us explore whether depressive and anxiety symptoms reached clinical or diagnosable levels. One meta-analysis synthesizing results of 28 studies comparing those with and without PCOS found that differences in depression and anxiety were moderate in size and more indicative of mild depressive symptoms (Veltman-Verhulst et al., 2012). By contrast, in a more recently published systematic review of 30 studies (18 of which were subjected to meta-analysis), results revealed higher risk in those with PCOS compared with those without (3–5 times greater likelihood, respectively, for depression and anxiety), and this risk reflected *moderate to severe* anxiety and depression (Cooney et al., 2017). Thus, evidence on clinical significance is mixed.

Even if symptoms do not reach clinically diagnosable levels, depression and anxiety experiences may still be meaningful in the lives of individuals living with PCOS. In the interviews that I conducted for the purpose of this book, I did not formally assess mental health symptoms and determine their severity. I did, however, ask individuals whether they experienced depression and anxiety. Among the 50 individuals I interviewed, 40 (80%) reported depression and 38 (76%) reported anxiety among their PCOS-specific symptoms. Although these percentages are high, they likely capture both those with formally diagnosed disorders and those with symptoms but no diagnoses. This broad approach may be helpful for the purpose here of understanding the lived experience of individuals rather than just those who have sought treatment to obtain a diagnosis, which may underestimate the psychological impact of PCOS.

Whether or not individuals with PCOS experience clinical levels of depression and anxiety, the quality of one's life can be compromised in the face of

PCOS. How is QOL determined? The World Health Organization (WHO; 1998) defines QOL as one's perceived position in life that considers contexts of one's culture and value system specifically in relation to one's expectations or goals, in multiple domains (e.g., physical, psychological, social, personal). Across multiple studies, research finds lower QOL scores in those with PCOS, relative to comparison groups (see Dokras et al., 2018, for a review). A 2011 meta-analysis combined the results of five studies from multiple countries, revealing that individuals with PCOS scored lower in QOL compared with individuals without PCOS who were matched on age (Li et al., 2011). Importantly, lower QOL is shown whether researchers use general QOL measures (e.g., Short Form Health Survey—36 [SF-36] or equivalent, which taps personal perceptions about physical, social, and emotional areas of life; Ware & Sherbourne, 1992) or PCOS-specific QOL based in PCOS symptom areas (e.g., body hair, weight, menstrual problems; Amiri et al., 2016; Cronin et al., 1998; Williams et al., 2018). Of note, some have critiqued PCOS-specific QOL measurements, qualifying that they may tap more into the personal impact of symptoms than QOL (Malik-Aslam et al., 2010).

Explanations for Increased Psychological Risk in PCOS

In sum, strong and accumulating evidence shows increased risk for major psychological outcomes of PCOS that include depression, anxiety, and lowered QOL. However, *why* are individuals with PCOS at such increased risk for negative psychological outcomes? There is not one robustly supported explanation in the research literature for these negative psychological outcomes among those with PCOS. What seems the most likely case is that a combination of PCOS and non-PCOS reasons explain risks. This lack of understanding of the cause of depression and anxiety in PCOS was echoed in the narratives of individuals I interviewed who simply did not know what role their PCOS played in their psychological outcomes. Some of their uncertainty about the role of PCOS in their depression and anxiety stemmed from a strong family history of mental health concerns or the simple fact that they always had dealt with depression and anxiety in their lives. These uncertainties are illustrated by the following excerpts.

> That's been . . . a lifelong struggle. . . . I don't . . . know how much of that . . . to attribute to PCOS. (*Emerson, mid-30s, nonbinary*)

> I feel like depression is . . . my baseline. I . . . feel like it's . . . my home. And then when I step out of that, it's . . . amazing. But I know I'm going to come back to it. (*Jonny, early 30s, nonbinary/transmasc*)

> I have always struggled with depression, since I was a child. And . . . I don't know how much that's related to the PCOS versus . . . me just being predisposed

> to depression. . . . I've experienced some trauma in my life, too. . . . But . . . it's something that when I look at the list of . . . symptoms of PCOS, it's one to . . . check off among many. (*Farah, mid-20s, nonbinary*)

In the remainder of this section, I describe the published research that has examined factors that predict increased psychological risk in PCOS to better understand why PCOS might be linked to such risk. I also present excerpts from my own interviews that support the particular explanation. Overall, this work underscores the need for future prospective or long-term studies on the multiple pathways that produce psychological risk to clarify how and why aspects of PCOS explain risk.

One line of research attempting to explain why PCOS is linked to psychological risk includes the direct role of biology related to hormones, insulin resistance, and obesity in those with PCOS (Barry, 2019). For example, some studies show insulin resistance or BMI as risk factors for depression, although the directionality of the relation is unclear (Greenwood et al., 2018, 2019). In addition, studies linking androgens such as testosterone to depression risk in PCOS are mixed, with some supporting a relation and some not (Dokras, 2012). Overall, these explanations do not completely account for the disparity in risk for depression and anxiety noted in the literature thus far (e.g., Dokras, 2012).

Some individuals I interviewed spoke directly about the link they perceived between hormones and their psychological symptoms. These comments reflected their lived experience of PCOS and what they noticed about the severity of their own symptoms in relation to depression and anxiety. For example, Jean noticed a link between hormones and psychological symptoms surrounding her menstrual cycles. Others described fluctuations in depression and anxiety based on how PCOS was medically treated with hormones. Emerson and Amy, for instance, noted differences from before to after treatment with birth control. Still others mentioned testosterone's impact specifically, such as Jack, who discussed high testosterone relating to psychological symptoms.

> I have more depression than I do anxiety. My anxiety is a lot more tied to situational factors. But my depression definitely is really, really connected to my hormones and really connected to however my cycle is going. . . . When I was younger, I struggled a lot with suicidal ideation and I realized once I got older that some of that—the timing of some of my worst bouts with it were connected to my cycle. (*Jean, late 20s, cisgender woman*)

> There were definitely times where . . . I was basically doing nothing to treat my PCOS and . . . mood and irritability was way worse. . . . on top of the anxiety and depression, . . . moodiness and . . . irritability . . . were really bad. (*Emerson, mid-30s, nonbinary*)

I've always kind of struggled with depression, but it really became prominent when I first was diagnosed with PCOS. They had put me on a type of birth control. . . . it completely tanked my mental health. I was having mood swings. I was . . . really impulsive. I would be talking to somebody and then all of a sudden, I'd get really angry. And the next minute I would just be . . . bawling my eyes out. And it was just really hard to . . . get up in the morning. And it was almost to the point that I was . . . becoming suicidal. And so I went back to them and told them to take me off this medicine that they had me on and we haven't tried the birth control thing since then. That's when . . . they put me on medicine for depression instead, and I'm no longer on any of the medications. But it [depression] still is like a pretty prominent part of my life. (*Amy, mid-20s, cisgender woman*)

My anxiety really spiked hard in my 20s, which when I look back also correlates with when some of my PCOS symptoms got a lot worse. . . . there were times where my mood would drop or my anxiety would peak in ways that . . . were just strange for me—very, very strange and unpredictable. The worst of it, I would say, was . . . about 5 years ago, right before I got diagnosed with PCOS . . . the doctor . . . did a bunch of testing and told me that I had PCOS and got me on metformin. . . . And one of the reasons that I had ended up going to a doctor that had an expertise in it was because I could not figure out what was wrong with my body. My periods were really, really intense. I was having—having some weird skin issues . . . the hair growth was really bad. Everything was really bad. And I couldn't figure out my mood. And when I went to her and she did the testing, she said that my hormones were so out of line with . . . what should be OK, that it was probably impacting my anxiety massively. And within 3 months of being on medication, all of a sudden, my mood had shifted completely. It was a very, very intense experience for me. (*Jack, mid-30s, nonbinary*)

Obesity associated with PCOS might also explain some of the risk for negative psychological outcomes, though it does not fully explain the psychological risk in those with PCOS (Dokras, 2012). In the most recent meta-analysis described earlier, even after examining only studies that had matched participants on BMI, risk for depression and anxiety was similarly high, indicating risk is not solely attributable to greater weight in those with PCOS relative to those without (Cooney et al., 2017). One recent study that used a longitudinal design tracked 163 individuals with PCOS over 5 years. Of the 59 originally screening positive for depression, obesity was a strong predictor of the depression persisting over the 5 years (Greenwood et al., 2019). As well, weight is among the strongest contributing factors to lower PCOS QOL regardless of the research method used (quantitative, Barnard et al., 2007; qualitative, G. L. Jones et al., 2011).

Many individuals with PCOS whom I interviewed also described associations between their weight gain or obesity and symptoms of depression and anxiety. Ricky specifically described the co-occurrence of weight gain and depression and anxiety. Cynthia mentioned a hopelessness attached to weight issues that continued despite her "doing all the right things." As Chapter 2 described, weight also brings about enacted and internalized stigma. Andi and Megan highlight the interconnectedness between weight-related stigma concerns and their psychological experiences with PCOS:

> When I was going through a period of time when it was an issue for me, I did gain a lot of weight, and I was experiencing a lot of more pain and that definitely— I definitely went through a period of depression and anxiety at that time. (*Ricky, early 40s, nonbinary*)

> When you're gaining weight really quickly and you're doing all the "right things" to not be gaining weight . . . it's really frustrating, because it's . . . a hopeless situation . . . I'm eating the right calories, I'm eating healthy carbs . . . no sugar or no alcohol. . . . And then, adding exercise on it, and it's sort of like, well, I can't create any more calorie deficit without becoming sick, so it's almost a hopeless feeling. . . . And, just the lack of confidence. I had a conference this summer that I was presenting [at] with . . . one of my colleagues . . . and I haven't seen him in years. I was like, oh my God, they're going to think I'm fat. People are taking our picture while we're talking. And . . . those sorts of things that just make me not want to be seen. (*Cynthia, mid-30s, cisgender woman*)

> The depression . . . kind of goes hand in hand with the weight gain and feeling like you won't fit in or being called names and things of that nature. And you just kind of feel down on yourself. Or, well, I would feel down on myself because I wasn't what people thought I should look like or even what I thought I should look like. So, depression would come in heavy. (*Andi, early 30s, cisgender woman*)

> The more . . . physical symptoms . . . have affected my mental health a lot, especially the weight . . . there are feelings of shame, kind of disgust with myself sometimes. When I don't exercise or when I just sit on the couch all day or if I read all day or sit on the couch or something, I feel bad because . . . I should have been exercising or doing something to get rid of the weight. So, I would say to . . . sum up, I think my mental health has been affected negatively. (*Megan, early 20s, cisgender woman*)

Hirsutism and acne also explain some but not all risks for depression and anxiety and lower QOL in PCOS. Recall from Chapter 1 that hirsutism (excess body hair) and acne are clinical indicators of PCOS-related hyperandrogenism. These can be associated with enacted and internalized stigma, as shown in Chapter 2. Hirsutism in particular, compared with multiple other PCOS symptoms, appears strongly predictive of anxiety (McCook et al., 2015). Associations between hirsutism and anxiety have been found in other studies in the United States and internationally (e.g., Italy; Borghi et al., 2018). Individuals I interviewed similarly linked their excess facial and body hair to their psychological symptoms of depression and anxiety. Farah implicated external factors of weight and body hair in depressive thoughts, whereas Cody specifically connected PCOS-related hair to anxiety. Jules made additional connections to the unfair treatment from others for reasons of their body hair as explaining depression and anxiety.

> I think the way that I look . . . experiencing facial hair and excess body hair growth and struggling with my weight has been something that's definitely . . . an environmental factor to my depression . . . I know I have . . . an imbalance of . . . chemicals in my brain, but I'm sure . . . external factors, too, and those are definitely . . . a part of my depressive thoughts . . . So, I would say it [PCOS] affects my mental health. (*Farah, mid-20s, nonbinary*)

> I admittedly . . . do suffer from both of those things [depression and anxiety] throughout my life. . . . the social impact [of PCOS] . . . it's excruciating and devastating on the mental health. . . . I was constantly being told to fix this, fix that . . . shave this, shave that. (*Jules, late 20s, nonbinary*)

> And depression and anxiety I struggle with, I don't know if it's because of the PCOS or if it's just because of me, but I have major depressive disorder . . . no matter what I do, I'm depressed. . . . I have felt a lot of anxiety in my life due to . . . the hair growth and the acne. I didn't mention acne before, but it was really bad for a while. And I experienced a lot of anxiety about my appearance . . . because of PCOS. (*Cody, mid-20s, nonbinary*)

Negative body image or body dissatisfaction stemming from external features of PCOS (e.g., hirsutism, obesity) may undergird negative psychological outcomes, also according to both prior research and the interviews I completed. We know that individuals with PCOS express greater body dissatisfaction in relation to body and facial hair as well as skin complexion and overall appearance relative to comparison groups (e.g., women with infertility but not PCOS; women with neither PCOS nor infertility; Himelein & Thatcher, 2006a). There also is evidence that body dissatisfaction contributes to negative psychological outcomes in those with PCOS. For example, one study found increased rates of anxiety and depression in PCOS and that body image distress fully explained the increased risk for these negative mental health outcomes (Alur-Gupta et al., 2019). The important role of body dissatisfaction in psychological outcomes in individuals with PCOS may call into question a sole focus on biological explanations for depression and anxiety (Himelein & Thatcher, 2006a). The central role of body dissatisfaction and external features of PCOS in QOL may be universally felt across cultures as well. For instance, an Iranian study of 300 women with PCOS from gynecological clinics revealed self-esteem and body image among the strongest explanations for lower health-related QOL (Bazarganipour et al., 2014), and a German study showed that BMI and hirsutism were the strongest contributors to physical QOL in 120 women with PCOS (Hahn et al., 2005). Individuals I interviewed described a link between their body image and depressive symptoms, particularly relating to weight and body hair.

> It makes it harder to view . . . myself [in] a positive light because of . . . being overweight and . . . the abnormal body hair. And it just takes its toll sometimes . . . especially . . . with depression . . . if you're having . . . a bad day . . . you go to take a shower, . . . get out of the shower and you look at yourself in the mirror and you just aren't happy with what you see. . . . And then you try to do things [to] make it better or . . . to change things, but it just doesn't come . . . easy—results . . . you would want. . . . So, it can make it really hard to keep a positive outlook. (*Amy, mid-20s, cisgender woman*)

PCOS-related body dissatisfaction as explanation for depression and anxiety risk makes sense given the stigmatizing nature of PCOS symptoms (see Chapter 2). Stigma can explain both the body dissatisfaction due to the physical characteristics of PCOS and why this dissatisfaction links with negative psychological outcomes (Wu & Berry, 2018). Body dissatisfaction itself has been described as a form of internalized weight stigma (Sikorski et al., 2015). In the context of weight, experiences of enacted stigma are related to more depression and anxiety, beyond what BMI itself might explain (Papadopoulos & Brennan, 2015). More generally, stigma impacts multiple factors of one's life that can explain negative psychological outcomes (Frost, 2011). One reason is that stigma-related stress can erode social, emotional, and coping resources that normally would help individuals cope during times of stress (e.g., Hatzenbuehler, 2009; Sikorski et al., 2015). Thus, the internalized and enacted stigma attached to PCOS symptoms that I discussed in Chapter 2 may further explain why psychological outcomes are worse in those with PCOS compared with those without.

Infertility is a common symptom of PCOS and one fraught with negative emotion and psychological risk (Chaudhari et al., 2018), especially given the stigmatizing nature of this symptom, as explained in Chapter 2. An additional contributing factor may be PCOS-related risk for pregnancy and delivery complications, especially when hyperandrogenism is experienced (beyond those attributable to obesity; Khomami et al., 2019). Yet variability in fertility goals may determine whether infertility status explains increased risk for psychological outcomes. Individuals living with PCOS whom I interviewed highlighted differing perspectives on infertility based on their fertility goals. Some individuals described depression due to infertility as well as fear of never having a child due to irregularity of menstrual cycles, whereas others feared pregnancy due to that same menstrual irregularity.

> I definitely experienced depression with the infertility. Because . . . everyone else was having kids with no problem. And here I . . . cannot . . . because of this freakin' PCOS and not ovulating. And it's like, "What do you mean I'm not ovulating? I'm a female." . . . it definitely makes you feel . . . less than. It does affect your womanhood—it does affect your womanhood. . . . You feel inadequate. You feel . . . less than. You feel like something is wrong with you.

I've even felt like, "Is God punishing me for something?"—you know, for my sins. It hits you physically, emotionally, mentally, spiritually and on every level, every aspect. This infertility . . . due to PCOS. And, you know, at times I was hiding. I would just go to work . . . and go home. I didn't even enjoy my summer. I was just inside, and I was just depressed. . . . Luckily for me . . . I only had to do one cycle of IVF [in vitro fertilization] . . . and luckily, God blessed me . . . with my son. . . . I always knew I wanted two children and then I thought I would have to go through another cycle of IVF. . . . And miraculously, I was able to conceive without in vitro. . . . I do, I feel blessed. . . . But I remember how I was feeling when I wasn't getting pregnant, when I was facing infertility issues. (*Valeria, early 40s, cisgender woman*)

The fear of not having children . . . it's definitely the fear of not being able to pass on a legacy. I literally just want one kid from my body. I'm adopting the rest. But I think that's . . . the biggest fear. Or to have a partner who wouldn't understand everything that could also come with PCOS. . . . Or having someone in my life who just doesn't get it. I don't know if that makes sense. . . . So, it affects my mental health because I feel like sometimes, . . . I'm somewhere and it's like holiday time. . . . I see a family together, and it will make me think, "OK, well, are you ever going to have that? Is that ever something that's going to be a part of you?" So, then I become depressed . . . so, my depression really stemmed . . . from thinking that I won't be able to have "the American dream." And that, I think, is the biggest thing, mental health wise . . . it kind of weighs on me. . . . The American dream . . . you got your house, your picket fence, your 2.5 kids. That's part of the American dream that was sold to us by Disney and everything. . . . having a family, and being fulfilled through that. That's kind of a thing that I'm always worried about. And that gets me further depressed, which will make me withdraw simply because . . . you're not good enough, that kind of attitude that comes in my brain. Stupid mush of meat. (*Andi, early 30s, cisgender woman*)

My period comes every . . . 32 days, but then it'll just not come . . . from 1 month it'll skip . . . up to like 6 months. . . . And oftentimes when it skips, I still get the PMS [premenstrual syndrome] and oftentimes PMDD [premenstrual dysphoric disorder] symptoms. But no menstrual cycle or no menstruation. And yes, I'll get all of the physical and emotional symptoms, but no actual blood. . . . It's really worrisome, because I am sexually active . . . especially before I knew that I had PCOS, it made me anxious all the time, even though I was using protection and I have IUD for a couple of years like I was—I was just always anxious that I was pregnant, which is actually kind of a phobia of mine. (*Jordan, late 20s, nonbinary/agender/sometimes woman*)

Other Underexplored Explanations

Still other PCOS-specific and non-PCOS explanations likely have an impact on risk for negative psychological outcomes in research. For example, although not yet examined in PCOS, individuals with diverse gender or racial/ethnic identity may have differing experiences of PCOS with unique implications for psychological outcomes. Limited research has considered racial/ethnic variation in PCOS-related mental health. One study, controlling for age, BMI, and socioeconomic status, showed significantly greater prevalence of anxiety in White compared with Black women with PCOS and no differences in depression or overall QOL (Alur-Gupta et al., 2021). As well, the information covered in Chapter 3 about the gendered embodiment of PCOS may be relevant here. These individuals encounter stigma attributable to their diverse gender and racial/ethnic identities, separate from PCOS. Greater understanding is needed on how PCOS and identity factors work together to influence psychological outcomes.

Another potential predictor of psychological risk in PCOS that deserves more attention is childhood or adult trauma. Some limited research shows a possible link between reports of adverse childhood experiences (ACEs) and psychological symptoms in individuals with PCOS (e.g., Tay et al., 2020). It is unclear at this time why individuals with PCOS might have an increased risk of exposure to adverse events in their childhood. At the very least, individuals living with PCOS who also have a trauma history may be additionally vulnerable to negative psychological outcomes. Experiencing ACEs in childhood challenges one's capacity to cope with other events, due to biopsychosocial changes brought on by early trauma (e.g., Winfrey & Perry, 2021).

Presumably, increased stress levels that result from all the preceding possible PCOS-related experiences could explain some increased psychological risk. It makes sense that stress may be elevated in individuals with PCOS given the range of symptoms they are dealing with, not to mention the potential for long-term chronic health conditions, such as diabetes and heart disease (to be discussed in Chapter 6). For example, in a recent community-based study of women's health in Australia, researchers found elevated levels of perceived stress in addition to elevated depression and anxiety in those with PCOS compared with individuals without (Damone et al., 2019). Furthermore, this perceived stress mediated or explained why PCOS was linked with elevated psychological outcomes. More research is needed on PCOS-related stress.

Thus, although more research has been conducted on psychological outcomes relative to other areas of psychosocial life addressed in this book, much more work is needed. Psychological risk for depression and anxiety and reduced QOL is apparent, but future research is needed that integrates the gamut of potential explanations for these negative psychological outcomes. This future work should simultaneously consider combinations of PCOS symptoms and explanatory factors to test comprehensively why individuals with PCOS are at increased risk (Bazarganipour et al., 2013). In addition to multiple PCOS symptoms and explanations, outcomes beyond depression, anxiety, and QOL need further investigation (e.g., bipolar disorder; Brutocao et al., 2018). One prime example is eating disorder risk. One meta-analysis of seven studies across five countries revealed individuals with PCOS are at a 3 times higher prevalence of eating disorder diagnosis and elevated disordered eating scores compared with those without (I. Lee et al., 2019). Binge eating disorder and bulimia nervosa in particular may be elevated among those with PCOS (I. Lee et al., 2017). Regrettably, I did not ask specifically about eating disorders in my interviews, and therefore eating-related issues were not typically discussed by individuals I interviewed. Regardless of the specific pathway through which PCOS influences psychological outcomes, it is evident that it takes a psychological toll on those living with the syndrome, as best summarized by a quote from Jaime, a genderfluid individual in her mid-30s: "It fucking hurts on so many levels—an emotional level, a physical level, a spiritual level. Energetically it hurts. It's not something that's easy."

PSYCHOLOGICAL GROWTH IN INDIVIDUALS LIVING WITH PCOS

The prior section summarized what we currently know about the risk of negative psychological outcomes and their potential explanations in individuals with PCOS. However, some individuals with PCOS may not experience negative psychological symptoms and may even grow in positive ways despite negative PCOS symptoms. Notably, any examination of positive psychological outcomes despite living with PCOS is completely absent from the published research on PCOS. Before exploring this possibility here, I begin with a couple of cautions. First, a focus on positive outcomes in PCOS should not negate or minimize the very real risk for negative psychological outcomes in PCOS like depression, anxiety, and reduced QOL. Second, discussion of positive outcomes should not add pressure to individuals living with PCOS to be positive. In other words, my intention is not to imply that individuals are somehow deficient if they do not report positive outcomes. With those cautions in mind, I discuss how individuals might grow in positive ways despite the challenges of PCOS in the hope that this information might benefit individuals living with PCOS. As well, psychological growth stemming from PCOS experience contributes new knowledge to research on PCOS.

I was taken aback by individuals' descriptions of positive outcomes despite or even *because of* having PCOS during the interviews. I recall having an internal emotional reaction to hearing one of my interviewees describe gratitude for PCOS because it had taught her so much about herself. Until that point, I was familiar with only the negative side of PCOS. Importantly, I noticed that individuals with this type of positive view of PCOS often described it as resulting from their journey of moving from negative experiences, such as extremely negative body image or shame, to acceptance. The word *journey* stood out because it reflected a process by which individuals began to make sense of or find meaning from their negative PCOS experiences and developed into a sense of empowerment detached from the societal expectations and shame about their bodies. Kim's excerpt that follows illustrates psychological growth present in the lives of the individuals I interviewed. She vividly described the simultaneous experience of many negative psychosocial impacts of PCOS discussed in this book—and also a gratitude for the diagnosis. This gratitude reflected a reframing of the PCOS diagnosis and experiences that displayed how she made positive meaning and grew from the negative experiences.

> PCOS has been a double-edged sword for me. In some ways it's been a gift, because it's pushed me to learn so much and accept so much about myself and my body. And, so, in that way . . . it's been a growth experience in a good way for me. I think that it's also caused distress because of the symptoms and because of the way that I sometimes get treated in a world. And so, I think that it really has . . . changed my life. I mean . . . obviously, it's part of my life. But . . . there are definitely times that I felt really broken. . . . Women get socialized to be mothers . . . and I have . . . a lot of grief about the fact that it would be difficult for me to be a biological parent. . . . My partner and I have decided that we're not going to do that. I grieve. . . . We get told . . . an essential function of being a woman is to have a baby. And so, I experienced a lot of sadness around the thought of not ever being pregnant. I have experienced a lot of sadness about being treated the way I do for my body size or that . . . sometimes I get teased about having facial hair. I also don't think I would trade that . . . trade having PCOS. I don't think that I would—I would take it away, because I have learned so much about myself through the process that has been invaluable that I wouldn't want to give that up. So, I feel like it's just affected my life, . . . in really profound ways . . . both harmful and helpful. . . . I feel like it's been helpful for me to understand how PCOS is affecting my body, so I don't . . . feel like I fight my body in negative ways anymore. I don't feel like I'm trying to be angry or hurtful. I definitely experienced disordered eating when I was younger . . . because of my body size, and I think that coming to understand my condition helped me to be comfortable in the body that I have . . . and be grateful, sounds sort of reductive, but . . . I'm grateful for my body as it is, and . . . doing the best [I] can to love my body. (*Kim, mid-30s, cisgender woman*)

Because no prior work exists on psychological growth or related positive outcomes in PCOS, I drew from the broader psychological literature to understand these findings. The process of psychological growth described in PCOS closely resembled the related concepts of *posttraumatic growth, benefit finding,* and *meaning making*. Let me take this opportunity to unpack these terms first before making the connections to PCOS. Posttraumatic growth involves positive changes in one's personal and social life (e.g., self, relationship with others, life philosophy) as a result of those adverse or stressful circumstances (Tedeschi & Calhoun, 1996, 2014). You may be thrown by the word *traumatic* in posttraumatic growth in relation to PCOS. To be clear, I would argue that PCOS is not itself a traumatic event but that the symptoms and outcomes of PCOS can be considered stressful. Therefore, I retained the broader phrasing of *psychological growth*.

One might show psychological growth due to finding benefits in stressful experiences. Benefit finding is similar to posttraumatic growth and is seen as a specific means of coping with stress rather than the psychological outcome of the stress (Helgeson et al., 2006; Martz & Livneh, 2016). For example, individuals with chronic illness conditions like multiple sclerosis (Mohr et al., 1999), cancer, and lupus (Katz et al., 2001) can derive benefits from the experience of their illness, including an appreciation for life and compassion for others' circumstances. Such benefit finding can be associated with more positive and less negative psychological outcomes (Helgeson et al., 2006; Katz et al., 2001). Aligned with both benefit finding and psychological growth, those I interviewed described the positive changes of realizing one is stronger than originally thought and having compassion for other people experiencing hardships. Excerpts by Jaime and Josie illustrate.

> I'm going to work to do my best with my best, but I'm also going to love this skin that I'm in. And it really has become less of a battle and more of an embracing of who I am right now and trying to be better, but still loving who I am right now and not really worrying about weight on the scale. . . . I think that PCOS has made me a stronger person, I guess. I'm going to pull out the positive from it. (*Jaime, mid-30s, genderfluid*)

> I know what it feels like to not have someone understand what you're going through. And I'm more . . . sensitive to other people's issues. I feel like I'm more compassionate or empathetic because you never really know what someone's going through, because PCOS you can't really see and other illnesses you also can't see. So, . . . I'm more compassionate. (*Josie, early 20s, cisgender woman*)

Psychological growth among individuals I interviewed reflected a process of deriving meaning from their PCOS experiences. Making meaning from one's stressful experiences generally is a process that reduces the discrepancy (and the distress that follows) between how a person appraises the stress (e.g., that it is unfair) and their beliefs about how the world works (the world is fair; Park, 2010). Having a medical condition, like PCOS, can challenge global beliefs of how the world works and our role in it, providing an opportunity for making meaning from the experience and even experiencing growth (Park, 2009, 2013). When emotional life experiences instigate a change in the ways we think about ourselves and our worlds, personal transformation can result (Tedeschi & Calhoun, 2012). Although people can make meaning in many ways, one of those ways is through acceptance (Evers et al., 2001), which was reported by individuals with PCOS whom I interviewed. Rather than acceptance of the need to adapt to the chronic condition of PCOS specifically (Evers et al., 2001), the narratives often referred to acceptance of oneself and one's bodily characteristics that are a consequence of PCOS.

Specifically, the positivity described by individuals living with PCOS reflected a movement from shame regarding one's PCOS symptoms or body to acceptance. This acceptance seemed to entail a turning point of coming to accept that PCOS symptoms are just a part of who they are. This acceptance is illustrated in the following excerpts by Kim, Marsh, and Dylan.

> I think that it's [mental health] improved over time, not just because of having . . . pharmacological help with medicine, but . . . I've also . . . learned to be unashamed about it because it's a condition that . . . is not changeable. It's just my body . . . I've felt less isolated and less depressed, less anxious about it because I feel like I've come to just accept my . . . body for who I am and . . . what it does for me and what it sometimes doesn't do for me. . . . I feel like I've been on a journey of growing towards better mental health as it relates to PCOS. But I definitely experienced depression, anxiety . . . at pretty high levels early on, until I felt like I had a name for what was going on, and . . . then . . . recently ways to manage the symptoms that are manageable. (*Kim, mid-30s, cisgender woman*)

> So, at this point, it's sort of it's like it's . . . an Instagram hashtag and it's just it's another part of me and who I am . . . it's . . . weirdly an important part of me because it's this diagnosis that has changed my body significantly and impacted my way of walking through the world. But it's not . . . like a negative diagnosis to me. It's been sort of like . . . an identity. (*Marsh, mid-30s, nonbinary*)

> The primary step in . . . that journey for most people is coming to terms with the fact that they have a good body, period. And it's from that . . . place that you're actually able to then think about food to fuel, to think about movement as a place of joy and expression and makes you feel good instead of . . . exercise for punishment. But it . . . for me and for others . . . centered on "there's nothing wrong with you" and . . . being able to internalize [that] . . . "you have a body that is good." (*Dylan, late 20s, genderqueer*)

This process of acceptance involved recognition of societal discrimination against bodies that violated expectations and a letting go of those societal expectations for oneself. At times this acceptance felt like resolve to not let negativity continue. Excerpts by Cody and Farah illustrate.

> It used to really bring me down and I used to feel a huge disconnect from my body . . . because of pressure from the rest of society. But as soon as I was able to let go of that pressure from society, now I really embrace my body and embrace my uniqueness and my differences. And I don't feel like I have to conform to anybody's box. And I'm really happy . . . the way that I am now. But it didn't always feel that way. (*Cody, mid-20s, nonbinary*)

> I think if I was younger . . . my answer would be my facial hair and my weight for sure, just because . . . I experienced bullying and . . . a lot of . . . emotional distress from having those symptoms. But . . . as I've gotten older and just come to . . . accept that these aren't things that can just go away. . . . I have to . . . move forward and find a way to be happy . . . those symptoms aren't as distressing to me as they used to be. (*Farah, mid-20s, nonbinary*)

The ability to extract positive meaning or growth from PCOS likely is influenced by dimensions of the illness condition (Park, 2009) as well as social and macro influences (Bronfenbrenner, 1979) and should be explored in future research. For example, the more domains of life that are disrupted by an illness and how chronic the condition, the more growth opportunities that may be created (Park, 2009). As we have seen in this book, PCOS certainly affects multiple areas of psychosocial life. As well, social or macro influences on coping with PCOS became apparent in some of the interviews I conducted. One salient example discussed by individuals holding minoritized racial/ethnic identities dealt with racial and ethnic inequalities. Andi expressed what being a woman of color had taught her and how it had prepared her to deal with a lot of injustices, including PCOS:

> I can't be mad at my body for doing what it decided to do. I could be slightly upset, but where is that going to get me in the long run? Where do I want to put my energy? . . . What do I want to be sad about today? It's kind of . . . my takeaway . . . having a good knowledge of yourself, and . . . accepting the things you can't change . . . I can never change my skin color. Unfortunately, I'm going to deal with racism my entire life. I hope that in two generations, we won't have that issue anymore . . . but being a [racial/ethnic identity] woman in America has helped me to come to terms with a lot of things or injustices or . . . slights that I feel. It's given me better coping mechanisms and better skills to be able to say, "OK, well, this isn't going to be the straw that breaks the camel's back today." (*Andi, early 30s, cisgender woman*)

I have not seen this type of critical analysis of social context within PCOS research. Researchers wanting to take a critical social lens to PCOS might learn from other areas of psychology already doing this work. For instance, researchers studying PCOS could learn from psychologists and others working with clients from marginalized groups and how they acknowledge the impact of oppression (e.g., racism, sexism) and root interventions in such ecological reality (Bartholomew et al., 2018). Racism is a unique form of stress that influences coping with other stress (e.g., Peters & Massey, 1983). At the same time, oppressed individuals, such as people of color, are activists in their own lives and resist such oppressions (Bartholomew et al., 2018). Applying these ideas, PCOS research should simultaneously examine the negative effects of PCOS and the psychological growth possible in the face of them.

In sum, individuals with PCOS experienced psychological growth in their lives despite or even *because of* PCOS. These experiences should be examined more systematically in future psychological research. As with psychological risk, it would be helpful to discern what factors contribute to this psychological growth in individuals living with PCOS. Admittedly, not everyone I interviewed discussed making meaning or finding psychological growth from their PCOS experiences. Furthermore, when individuals did report psychological growth, they emphasized words like *journey* to denote that movement from shame to acceptance did not happen quickly but rather was a process that took time. Thus, growth may be one of several potential outcomes and may take time to develop (Helgeson et al., 2006).

CONCLUSION

This chapter presented evidence from published research on PCOS, combined with excerpts from interviews I conducted, that individuals with PCOS are at risk for negative psychological outcomes such as depression, anxiety, and lower QOL. A number of potential explanations for those risks exist that need further investigation, knowing that it is likely a combination of PCOS-specific and non-PCOS factors that simultaneously contribute. Finally, this chapter broke new ground by describing psychological growth experiences that individuals living with PCOS personally cultivated through journeys toward self-acceptance. Despite the real struggles involved with PCOS, there may also be opportunities to discover personal strength and acceptance. Such psychological growth seems especially valuable for coping with a lifelong condition that has no known cure. In the next chapter, I explore physical health risks of PCOS and individuals' experiences with health care.

6 HEALTH RISKS AND INADEQUATE PCOS HEALTH CARE RESOURCES

How can we step outside this culture enough to see a path forward where demanding social support for our biology is a feminist act? . . . There's only so much we can ask of our bodies.

–Jennifer Block (2019, pp. 282-283), *Everything Below the Waist: Why Healthcare Needs a Feminist Revolution*

Chapter 5 presented evidence that many individuals living with polycystic ovary syndrome (PCOS) experience negative psychological outcomes and, at the same time, that they may grow in positive ways from challenges of the syndrome. In addition to psychological outcomes, PCOS also has implications for major health outcomes, thereby implying the importance of available quality PCOS health care. This sixth chapter of the book investigates PCOS-specific health care experiences among individuals living with PCOS, showing the inadequacy of available PCOS health care resources. As with prior chapters, Chapter 6 highlights unique challenges of diverse groups seeking PCOS health care, underscoring the need to improve cultural competence among health care providers. Health risks and health care experiences are directly relevant

https://doi.org/10.1037/0000337-007
The Psychology of PCOS: Building the Science and Breaking the Silence, by S. L. Williams

for building a psychological science of PCOS, given the interconnectedness between physical and mental health and between health care and mental health care. These interconnections are further addressed in the next chapter on improving PCOS-related health care and mental health interventions.

PHYSICAL HEALTH RISKS AND COMPLICATIONS OF PCOS

This chapter describes individuals' experiences with PCOS-specific health care as yet another way that PCOS affects psychosocial aspects of their lives. This topic is relevant because individuals with PCOS are at increased risk for major chronic health conditions and are more likely to enter the health care system than those without PCOS (Hart & Doherty, 2015). Those with PCOS appear to be at increased risk for obesity, diabetes, cardiovascular disease, dyslipidemia (high cholesterol), hypertension (high blood pressure), fatty liver disease, endometrial cancer, and a compilation of symptoms known to increase risk for cardiovascular disease and diabetes known as metabolic syndrome (Azziz, 2018). Several of these are the major health conditions of our modern time. The statistics in these areas actually suggest not just risk but *sizeable* risk, such as a sevenfold increased risk of heart attack (Carmina & Lobo, 1999) and an 11-fold greater risk of developing metabolic syndrome (Dokras et al., 2005). Incidence of metabolic syndrome also may be higher in Black individuals with PCOS compared with White individuals, according to a recent longitudinal study (I. Lee et al., 2022). However, metabolic risk may be lower in those with PCOS characterized by symptoms of menstrual irregularity and polycystic ovaries but not hyperandrogenism (Shroff et al., 2007) and in lean PCOS (Lim et al., 2019). Recall from Chapter 1 that hyperandrogenism in PCOS involves excess testosterone with clinical symptoms of hirsutism, acne, and scalp hair loss. These long-term morbidities associated with PCOS contribute significantly to the economic health care burden of PCOS on society discussed in Chapter 1, which is estimated at $8 billion per year in the United States alone (Riestenberg et al., 2022).

Another alarming reason for the relevance of this topic is that despite the seriousness of these health risks, they have not been prioritized in health care, presumably because of the continued focus on the reproductive aspects of PCOS. To provide a personal example, I have had PCOS for more than 30 years. In my 3 decades' worth of health care visits, I have never had a health care provider tell me that my PCOS puts me at increased risk for other chronic conditions. To boot, I recently asked my general practitioner for suggestions of specialists with expertise in PCOS, to seek guidance on how

I might optimize my health to avoid these health impacts (if that is possible). She assured me that because I was not interested in reproduction, there was no need for a specialist or other information on PCOS. As you might imagine, I was not assured.

In part, this lack of prioritization is because of limited long-term health studies with large samples of individuals with PCOS. In fact, my general practitioner cited this lack of research findings in her response to me about there being no evidence of needing specialized care. A systematic review of the literature on long-term risk in reproductive- and older-age (above 40) women with PCOS confirmed the need for large cohort studies assessing risk starting in reproductive age and prospectively into old age—which is when risk for chronic conditions increases independent of PCOS (Cooney & Dokras, 2018). Whereas PCOS symptoms themselves may improve with age (more regular menstruation, later menopause), the long-term impact on chronic diseases into old age is lesser known (Hoeger et al., 2021). Additionally, any available data associating PCOS with chronic health conditions come solely from patients referred to treatment (Lizneva et al., 2016). In other words, the sampling bias (e.g., participants are clinic-based) previously discussed may limit complete understanding of long-term outcomes of PCOS. Finally, limited PCOS research specifies health risks and health care utilization in diverse groups based on gender and racial/ethnic identity. Meanwhile, there are plenty of data to support health disparities—or the systematic and worse health outcomes experienced by minoritized racial/ethnic and gender identity groups and those of low socioeconomic status (National Academies of Science, Engineering, and Medicine, 2017).

Importantly, lack of research funding may largely undergird the lack of long-term research on PCOS. A comparison of National Institutes of Health funding between PCOS and conditions with similar or lower prevalence, morbidity, and mortality (rheumatoid arthritis, tuberculosis, and lupus) revealed that not only did PCOS research receive relatively less funding but that fewer institutes were involved in that funding—only one institute (the National Institute of Child Health and Human Development, which is focused on reproductive health) funded PCOS research (Brakta et al., 2017). Given the actual burden of PCOS (economic, quality of life, morbidity), these findings indeed support the notion that PCOS research is underfunded relative to other conditions. There is a clear imperative for funding agencies to prioritize PCOS research and for researchers to identify long-term risks and who is most vulnerable to them.

Returning to the main point, investigating the health care experiences of individuals living with PCOS would speak to the lack of availability of quality health care for managing a condition that puts them at risk for health problems and increased need for health care. In this chapter, I describe health care experiences reported by the individuals living with PCOS whom I interviewed, combined with findings of prior research where available. As you will see, the health care system often does not meet the needs of individuals in need of diagnosis or treatment. Instead, experiences with PCOS health care reflect an overall dissatisfaction among patients due to providers' lack of knowledge about PCOS, delayed diagnostic experiences, and poor interactions with providers, all of which highlight ways health care must be changed to improve patient experience.

DISSATISFACTION WITH HEALTH CARE

The vast majority (more than 90%) of those I interviewed described dissatisfaction with health care in the context of various PCOS-specific symptoms and treatment. The paragraphs that follow illustrate a range of encounters that also represent themes previously identified in prior PCOS-specific health care research (lack of knowledge, delayed diagnosis, dismissive responses; Crete & Adamshick, 2011; Soucie et al., 2021; Tomlinson et al., 2017) and non-PCOS health care research (weight bias, lack of cultural competence). Importantly, these narratives also highlight the areas where health care could be reformed to improve PCOS-specific health care, which I introduce in the next chapter.

Lack of Provider Knowledge of PCOS

One conclusion we can draw about PCOS health care is that many health care providers lack appropriate knowledge about PCOS. For example, a 2007 survey assessed knowledge, comfort, and referral behaviors related to two women's health topics (menopause and PCOS) and two gender-neutral health concerns (diabetes, thyroid disease) among 50 medical residents, 36 of which were part of a women's health track designed to help improve their training (Spencer et al., 2007). Although residents, on average, scored 50% on PCOS knowledge (recognition of clinical presentation, diagnostic workup), only 44% of those with women's health training and 23% of those without got more than 70% of the information correct. PCOS-specific knowledge scores were the lowest out of all four health concerns examined.

Importantly, patients recognize this lack of knowledge. Indeed, more than half of the individuals I interviewed described lack of provider knowledge in their narratives. As illustrated by Abigail and Joni's excerpts, they were dismayed when providers were missing key information about PCOS and had to educate them:

> He's [provider's] like, "I didn't realize that . . . male pattern hair . . . was from PCOS. . . . I thought it [PCOS] was just ovarian cysts." And I'm like, "Well, you're going to be shocked to know that I don't even have ovarian cysts." (*Abigail, mid-20s, nonbinary*)

> I shouldn't have to educate my providers. If it's something that's . . . a rare issue, that would be understandable if doctors hadn't heard about it or didn't know about it, but PCOS is very common. I should not have to educate my providers on it. (*Joni, mid-20s, cisgender woman*)

When providers lack knowledge about PCOS, they cannot fully understand the symptoms their patients are experiencing. In a qualitative study of 20 individuals with PCOS and five health care providers, researchers discovered a discrepancy between patient and provider reports of what symptoms were important for those with PCOS (Martin et al., 2017). The study found providers did not identify heavy bleeding, cramping, and bloating as important to patients with PCOS, yet these were among the most frequently reported symptoms among patients.

The individuals living with PCOS whom I interviewed described how providers lacked knowledge about PCOS, which led to confusion about their own medical condition. For example, Emerson also dealt with thyroid disease and endometriosis and described that PCOS symptoms often "bleed into" these other conditions. The missing provider knowledge seemed particularly baffling to Emerson given the provider was an endocrinologist—and PCOS is an endocrine disorder.

> The health care industry in this country is very frustrating to deal with. . . . I've gone to see doctors about other things and like have had to explain PCOS to other doctors. . . . I had an endocrinologist that I saw for my thyroid disease that didn't know anything about PCOS. . . . I'm like, "How? . . . why am I having to educate you right now?" And . . . some of the symptoms can be kind of vague and they can bleed into other things . . . I also have endometriosis. . . . if you don't understand this [PCOS], then . . . you can't see how it overlaps with . . . anything else that's going on. . . . I just don't feel like I've ever had a doctor that could look at all my issues . . . holistically and with the understanding of PCOS and see how it is or isn't contributing to . . . whatever is going on with me at the time. (*Emerson, mid-30s, nonbinary*)

Angelina's provider assumed she had diabetes because she was taking a medication often prescribed to individuals with diabetes to treat her insulin resistance, which is part of PCOS (but does not equate to a diabetes diagnosis):

> It feels like a lot of people . . . even doctors . . . don't know what [PCOS] was. My . . . PCP came in the other day and she's like, "Hey, it looks like your diabetes

is under control." And I was like, "But am I diabetic? I'm not diabetic." . . . Because I was taking metformin. . . . "I'm not diabetic, am I?" (*Angelina, late 30s, cisgender woman*)

Delayed PCOS Diagnosis

The chasm between patient symptoms and provider knowledge of PCOS leads to delayed diagnosis of PCOS. Indeed, multiple large-scale quantitative studies have documented an unacceptable length of delay in the diagnosis process. One such study surveyed 210 community individuals with PCOS in Australia and found that it had taken a quarter of the individuals more than 2 years to receive a diagnosis of PCOS, and it had taken a third of the individuals visiting three health care providers before obtaining the diagnosis (Gibson-Helm et al., 2014). Delayed diagnosis is a global phenomenon, according to leading international researchers on PCOS. Similar findings emerged from their survey of 1,385 individuals with PCOS from 32 different countries across the globe; it took more than 2 years (for one third of the sample) and three or more health professionals (for nearly half of their sample) to receive a PCOS diagnosis (Gibson-Helm et al., 2017).

The individuals I interviewed spoke about their delayed diagnoses. Joni described the frustration of not getting a diagnosis until age 24, even though symptoms of PCOS were evident well before. Several others directly linked their delayed diagnosis to the lack of PCOS knowledge among providers. For example, Jonny received a diagnosis only after they learned about PCOS on their own and educated their health providers.

I've talked . . . with so many different providers [about] these issues and symptoms that I'm experiencing. And it took until I was 24, just years and years and years of so many different providers and specialists. And just now, very recently, had someone say, "Have you ever been checked for PCOS?" And so that's been frustrating for me because in hindsight, now that I know more about PCOS, . . . this makes perfect sense to me, now in hindsight. And, so, to have that . . . ignored for so long was . . . extremely frustrating for me. And then also finding out about the insulin resistance . . . that is a concern of mine. . . . Type 2 diabetes runs in my family, and so to never have anyone really . . . look into it, even though I have obvious symptoms, was also frustrating for me. (*Joni, mid-20s, cisgender woman*)

For as common as it [PCOS] is . . . the knowledge is not there. . . . My doctor that diagnosed me—I really had to push. . . . I had to talk to her about it on a couple of different occasions. And before that . . . I had said . . . I have this and this and this problem . . . I have amenorrhea or dysmenorrhea . . . my cycles are all messed up and I have hair and this and that. And . . . they didn't try to pursue it at all . . . had I not learned about PCOS, I probably still would not have a diagnosis. . . . I had to push for it. I had to pursue it . . . I just wish there was more knowledge. (*Jonny, early 30s, nonbinary/transmasc*)

Whereas delayed diagnosis occurs across patient demographic characteristics, issues of race or socioeconomic status may further exacerbate the health care challenges of PCOS. Although, to my knowledge, no studies have examined patient demographic characteristics as contributing to further delays in diagnosis, some literature points to implicit bias in health care, or subtle behaviors stemming from negative attitudes toward people of color that result in differential PCOS treatment (e.g., patient centeredness, diagnostic testing; Hall et al., 2015). Such bias in PCOS health care could translate into even bigger delays for PCOS patients representing other diverse identity groups. Among individuals I interviewed, Alia pointed to racial bias as contributing to delayed diagnosis of PCOS, and Janice underscored socioeconomic disparities in health information and PCOS health care.

There is something that has come up in groups [online PCOS-specific groups]. It's the issue of race. I have noticed that . . . there are Black women who get diagnosed very, very late, because . . . they're not believed probably for 10, 20 years. They have to have a cyst burst before they're believed. (*Alia, early 30s, cisgender woman*)

Where I grew up is a very lower educated area . . . my mom didn't have the best job, and we were low income and we would go to . . . the health department for our well checks . . . and we had doctors that were under Medicaid. . . . I know that this is an overgeneralized stereotype, but typically they don't seem to care as much. . . . I feel like our diagnoses were pushed off until we were older because I didn't get diagnosed [with PCOS] until I started going on my own when I was 19. And I feel like if I were educated about it earlier or if a physician had told me about it earlier, or even my sister, we could have a different outcome. Whether it be with weight management or depression or anxiety or stuff like that. I feel like we could have managed it better growing up, than kind of getting hit with it when we're starting out adult life and figuring everything else out on top of it. (*Janice, late 20s, cisgender woman*)

Expectedly, delayed diagnosis is associated with less satisfaction with the diagnostic process (Gibson-Helm et al., 2017). You can imagine that in addition to frustration surrounding suffering with unknown symptoms, delayed diagnosis can have larger implications for worse PCOS symptoms and health. During interviews, those with PCOS described life-altering implications of the diagnostic delay in their lives. Maria raised implications for her fertility. Specifically, she would have saved her eggs as a teenager if she had known infertility was her future. Tina believed her PCOS would not be as severe;

that is, perhaps the severity of the PCOS symptoms of insulin resistance and weight gain would have been less, and she would have had less shame for having the explanation of PCOS for facial hair. Of course, there may be other, longer-term implications of delayed diagnosis, considering that PCOS is associated with greater risk for major cardiovascular and metabolic problems over time. Any delay in getting diagnosed could have implications for such symptoms and, ultimately, life outcomes.

> Knowing that I had it early on would have saved me from so much more . . . later on in life . . . I feel that it would have given me a priority, if we're supposed to do . . . fertility treatments or not early on . . . save my eggs or . . . something early. . . . I got married later in life . . . close to my 30s . . . So, it would have been helpful knowing . . . as a teenager. . . . it would have helped me later on, whether it was saving my eggs or just taking more care of myself or just so many things. (*Maria, late 30s, cisgender woman*)

> If it hadn't been so long, I wouldn't have developed the insulin resistance, which, . . . caused the weight gain and yada, yada, yada. It's all snowballed. So, I think that getting doctors better training on this—I think it's really important. I think it would save people a lot of shame for those women who do grow facial hair. . . . knowing that's why. (*Tina, late 20s, cisgender woman*)

Poor Provider-Patient Interactions

In addition to lack of provider knowledge and delayed diagnosis, PCOS-related health care encounters are fraught with poor interactions between patients and providers. As described in this section, individuals living with PCOS characterized these interactions as dismissive and evidencing weight bias and cultural incompetence. These findings contribute to understanding of inadequate PCOS-specific health care experiences, particularly among individuals living with PCOS who represent other diverse groups.

Dismissive Responses From Providers

I am not the first to claim that health care providers are dismissive of PCOS symptoms and their patients' experiences (S. L. Williams et al., 2015). Dismissive behaviors from providers have been reported in the United States and other countries. For example, a group of researchers in Ontario, Canada, found PCOS patients' experiences in health care to include dismissive responses from providers, overall negative health care encounters, limited treatment options for PCOS (birth control as only option), a sense of uncertainty about the future due to the condition, and reliance on self-education often through reaching out to online and social media sources (Soucie et al., 2021). Similar themes were found in a U.S. study of women with PCOS in the mid-Atlantic region. Patients were frustrated with provider inattention to their symptoms, confusion due to lack of PCOS knowledge, their need for self-education through other sources of information such as the internet, and their own attempts to gain control over their own health through self-treatment (Crete & Adamshick, 2011).

These reports of dismissive behaviors from providers are common, as evidenced in the interviews with individuals living with PCOS. On the basis of their narratives, some of the dismissive behavior appeared to stem from treatment options that were one-size-fits-all or that reinforced norms or expectations that might not fit for individual differences in what people want. Other dismissiveness reflected providers' assumptions that PCOS is only a problem if someone wants to get pregnant. These examples are illustrated with excerpts from Cynthia, Asia, and Dylan.

> I think my health care experiences have been pretty poor. From being misdiagnosed for IBS [irritable bowel syndrome] at 22, and then even going on into being in the emergency room and just being told, "Oh, you're having a bad period." It has not all been male doctors. I will say that some of the female doctors have been pretty . . . clueless, too . . . a little bit dismissive of my concerns. (*Cynthia, mid-30s, cisgender woman*)

> I would say it's a mixture . . . there [are] days where . . . I will talk to different doctors and they will be understanding and have compassion and just listen to my concerns without judgment . . . There will be times where they will just be so dismissive . . . with the weight loss and everything. It's always "lose weight, do this, do that, eat healthier, be confident, . . . treat your depression." . . . They don't seem to want to get it. They don't listen, and they lack empathy. They . . . have no . . . compassion whatsoever for what I'm going through. (*Asia, mid-20s, cisgender woman*)

> When . . . expressing concern to a gynecologist . . . about my menstruation and lack of ovulation, she said, "Well, do you want to have kids?" I said, "No." She said, "Well, then it really doesn't matter, and there's always IVF [in vitro fertilization]." She flippantly responded that IVF was the treatment, as though IVF was a very simple walk in the park. And I was floored and appalled, and I never saw her again. . . . Over the course of my experience with PCOS, I have learned how to fire doctors. I've gotten really good at never coming back in, refusing treatment and telling them what I would like to have happen. I've had to get really ardent and defensive about my medical care and have had to do a ton of research to find . . . physicians and . . . people in medical professions who would be able to treat me with the respect that I deserve. (*Dylan, late 20s, genderqueer*)

Being dismissed by providers may be akin to medical "gaslighting," or the dismissal of patients to the point they begin to doubt themselves (Hand, 2021). Although no one I interviewed directly used the word "gaslighting" in context of providers, one individual reported a self-gaslighting that can happen when one questions their own symptoms as a result of lack of medical information and understanding. At the very least, this topic needs to be explored further in research, along with research on dismissive behaviors more generally.

> You check off . . . eight out of 10 symptoms, but there's no . . . test that . . . can definitely diagnose you. It's something that . . . is really frustrating and can then cause you to . . . feel like there's no closure . . . I may then gaslight myself . . . not knowing what symptoms are from PCOS and what aren't . . . is this an excuse for the fact that I'm fat and . . . it's hard for me to lose weight? . . . everything being so unclear and . . . uncertain is . . . really frustrating. And then . . . you're encouraged to go on birth control to . . . regulate things, but . . . there isn't . . . an actual . . . cure. It's just . . . managing symptoms. . . . And there isn't . . . a true diagnosis either . . . I think . . . it's my own fault that I'm having these symptoms . . . because I don't have confirmation that I even . . . have PCOS. . . . It can be . . . your own fault that you're . . . fat and have skin tags and . . . high cholesterol and are depressed. And then . . . a voice in my head [is] saying . . . I actually have PCOS . . . that makes these things more extreme or . . . causes these things. But it's hard to actually believe that when it feels like there's no solid evidence of it. (*Loren, early 20s, nonbinary*)

Weight Bias

Individuals living with PCOS commonly experienced weight bias in health care interactions. *Weight bias,* or the negative attitudes and discrimination toward individuals classified as overweight or obese, occurs in many contexts (Puhl & Brownell, 2001). Recall that in Chapter 2, I described this bias as weight stigma that occurs in multiple contexts. In research on health care the term *bias* is often used to represent weight stigma experiences. Although no published research has yet documented weight bias in health care as a problem for individuals with PCOS, ample evidence exists more generally to support this type of bias happening. Providers often hold the assumption that thin bodies are healthy, and fat bodies are unhealthy (Webb & Quennerstedt, 2010). They attribute any health problems in overweight patients to their weight (Alberga et al., 2019; Jímenez-Loaisa et al., 2020), act in disrespectful ways toward overweight patients, and attribute patient weight gain to poor diet and poor health behaviors (Alberga et al., 2019; Ananthakumar et al., 2020). Providers assume overweight patients eat unhealthy or "junk" food and do not exercise, which leads to ubiquitous advice from physicians for patients to eat less and exercise more (Ananthakumar et al., 2020).

Evidence of this weight bias in individuals living with PCOS I interviewed was found in their reports of providers' sole focus on their weight and weight loss during the health care visit. This focus reflected an assumption that weight is a patient's main or only problem and therefore that weight loss is the only solution, even though it merely "skirts around" the real issue of PCOS, as Dylan described:

> The recommendations for weight loss and for birth control as a primary treatment were really unsatisfactory and feel like they completely skirted around what's going on . . . [and] caused harm to reinforce that like, my body size needs to change in order for this to be "better" in the way that they think that "better" works. That's been really hard. (*Dylan, late 20s, genderqueer*)

The weight loss recommendation is especially challenging given that the very condition of PCOS makes it harder to lose weight. Providers fail to acknowledge this inherent challenge, which then results in perceived blame and shame from providers that individuals caused their own PCOS or weight. Excerpts from Farah, Leah, and Zoe illustrate their experiences of bias toward weight loss without recognition of PCOS from their health care providers.

> He [doctor] often . . . will bring up my weight as an issue and something I need to work on and . . . never has talked about it in the context of PCOS. . . . I feel uncomfortable to bring it up to him and feel like I'm making an excuse for myself. And that's definitely really uncomfortable for me, something I wish would change. And . . . I'm not really sure what to do about it. (*Farah, mid-20s, nonbinary*)

> We haven't really come up, as far as I know, with any good treatments in the entire time that I've been diagnosed with PCOS, which has been 25 years. In the meantime, every doctor that I've had shamed me about my weight and tells me to lose weight. Even though they know that it's virtually impossible for me to do because I have PCOS, they still tell me to do it. (*Leah, mid-40s, cisgender(ish) woman*)

> I grew up fat. I've seen many nutritionists in my life . . . it's funny because . . . fat people actually know more about nutrition than thin people do because most of us have been forced to see a nutritionist. . . . I do enjoy fruits and veggies. But I think something else is going on here . . . it's not just that . . . It has been a journey to finding—to finding good health care around PCOS. . . . It took forever for me to be diagnosed because it was always "just lose weight, just lose weight, just lose weight and you'll get your period." (*Zoe, late 20s, genderqueer*)

The intense focus on weight in health care can have harmful implications related to disordered eating or recognizing disordered eating. Ginna described an interaction with a provider who suggested that it was fine to restrict calories to the level of an eating disorder to lose weight. Joni shared that she had an eating disorder that involved exercising three times a day but that her provider suggested she exercise *more* as a means to lose weight.

Jo described paranoia about gaining weight that had been reinforced in health care. Leah described an interaction with a nutritionist who did not believe that she did not binge eat at night.

> [At] my very last doctor's appointment that I had, I was telling my doctor that I was struggling to lose weight, and I was wondering if we could up my . . . metformin. And he said he didn't really want to up the metformin right now, but maybe I could just control my diet better. And I was like, "Well, I already restrict calories. There are some days where I don't eat more than three or five hundred calories a day, and I know that's not healthy." And, he's like, "Well, that's OK." . . . So, you end up internalizing that . . . it's your fault . . . I need to eat less. I need to work out more. But no matter what you do, it doesn't change. (*Ginna, mid-30s, cisgender woman*)

> In the health care field, there's a lot assumptions . . . automatically assuming that my diet is very poor, that I don't exercise, or that I don't take care of myself, that I'm lazy, those types of things. . . . I've definitely had providers say things like, "you just need to exercise more" and . . . that's a big component of my eating disorder. So sometimes, I'm like, "I'm already exercising three times a day. What more do you want from me?" (*Joni, mid-20s, cisgender woman*)

> I've never been in a larger body and I don't think that there's anything wrong with being in a larger body. I very much believe in . . . body liberation and fat positivity. But I've also had an eating disorder for most of my life. . . . I guess [I have] paranoia about needing to make sure that I don't gain weight at any point, and that's sort of been enforced by how doctors have talked to me about having PCOS, like "Make sure you don't gain any weight." I saw one gynecologist nurse, like, "What do you think I should do about PCOS?" and she was like, "Well, you're fine because you're thin." And that's terrible. (*Jo, late 20s, genderqueer/nonbinary*)

> My first OBGYN experience was . . . incredibly, incredibly painful. And they told me, at the time, that the reason it was painful was because I was fat . . . blaming me for my genital pain. So that was certainly one of my negative PCOS health experiences. . . . Then, I went to college. I remember the college health center. They were like, "You're really big. We really think that you should see the nutritionist." So, I go to see the nutritionist and the nutritionist is like, "When you wake up in the middle of the night and binge, what do you binge on?" And I was like, "OK . . . I've never done that." And she was like, "I don't believe you." (*Leah, mid-40s, cisgender(ish) woman*)

Because individuals had experienced weight bias in health care, they anticipated poor treatment in future encounters and therefore avoided health care, as illustrated by Ginna's and Jack's excerpts. This fear of anticipated poor treatment from providers is reminiscent of vigilance for unfair treatment that disadvantaged groups experience when interacting with members of advantaged groups (Major et al., 2013).

There's been times where I don't want to go to the doctor, because I'm afraid they're going to harp on the weight or things that I don't really feel like I can control as well all by myself. (*Ginna, mid-30s, cisgender woman*)

When I look back at . . . old OBGYNs of mine . . . I've had so many [OBGYNs] . . . dismiss stuff and immediately take it to my weight that I, like a lot of other fat folks, . . . just stopped going to the doctor for a long time, which probably did not help . . . my medical issues. . . . But the reason I didn't go was because I felt totally overlooked and dismissed by everybody I talked to. . . . I can't believe how many times . . . I've gone in and told doctors about stuff that . . . now I look back [was] probably something with PCOS . . . bad pain, periods . . . and . . . they would still turn to weight loss. I'd be like, "Oh my gosh, are you even listening to me right now?" . . . I actually [had] real serious disdain . . . for medical doctors for a long time. And when my anxiety would peak . . . I was scared of them. I was scared to be dismissed and I was scared to be not heard. (*Jack, mid-30s, nonbinary*)

Weight bias in health care may not only be common but inadvertently legitimized given that lifestyle management is considered best practice in medical care of PCOS patients (Teede et al., 2018). That is, weight loss is the go-to strategy for managing PCOS given that there is no known cause and therefore no cure. This best practice may actually contribute to patients' perception that providers harbor weight bias and treat them based on unfair assumptions. Whereas providers may be implementing a best practice by offering lifestyle management advice intended to help patients manage PCOS symptoms, this advice is registered among patients as weight bias from the provider. Thus, at the very least, there is incongruence between provider intent and patient perception that needs addressed, to reduce the impact of weight bias (see Chapter 7).

Lack of Cultural Competence

The weight-based bias among providers may be symptomatic of a larger problem related to poor cultural competence in working with diverse patient populations. Although cultural incompetence has not yet been documented in PCOS patients, a long line of research evidences racism and gender bias in health care more generally. In 2003, the Institute of Medicine reported that bias, prejudice, and stereotypes, combined with medical uncertainty, can contribute to racial/ethnic disparities for people of color in health care (in other words, worse experiences systematically found in minoritized groups). Multiple reviews of the published literature show racism among health care providers as well (Paradies et al., 2014), with patient reports of worse health care satisfaction and communication linked to that racism (Ben et al., 2017).

Thus, negative PCOS-related health care encounters among people of color may be further attributable to racism. While the direct or explicit forms of bias may have diminished in recent years, implicit bias—the unconscious negative attitudes that individuals hold toward non-White individuals—remains. Unconscious bias toward people of color can be expressed in provider behaviors such as tone of voice, more or less diagnostic testing, and differential treatment recommendations (Hall et al., 2015). A systematic review of literature revealed low to moderate levels of implicit bias against people of color by health care providers (Hall et al., 2015). These unconscious biases are especially insidious because they impact provider–patient interactions; meanwhile, because of their implicit nature, they remain outside of provider awareness, making them difficult to change.

The individuals with PCOS whom I interviewed described experiencing race-based cultural insensitivity from their providers that also combined with bias about gender and weight to influence their treatment experience. The illustrative excerpts provided here are from two individuals of color with different gender identities. Both excerpts referenced ubiquitous racism, implying the need to advocate for oneself in healthcare because of it.

> I think a lot of providers need to check their fatphobia and racism that they might not even notice they have . . . those things . . . get in the way of me receiving nonjudgmental care and for a bunch of . . . people close to me that . . . have PCOS, some of them are also nonbinary or . . . trans men and some of them are fat, and they've all had less than stellar experiences with health care providers because of all these things. . . . sometimes doctors just tell you, "OK, well, lose weight" and they don't go into causes or . . . try to figure out what's going on with you, whether it's because you're a woman of color or a fat woman of color . . . I think we're just very easily dismissed. So that definitely impacted how long it took to get my diagnosis, to get treatment, to even realize it myself. (*Riley, early 20s, nonbinary*)

> Doctors tend not to . . . take [racial/ethnic identity] women's health seriously. Like they always brush us off. It . . . happens to me and it happens to other [racial/ethnic identity] women. And I just feel like that's something important because racism in health care is very obvious and it happens a lot. And I feel like people need to know more about it . . . different studies . . . show that [racial/ethnic identity] women don't get taken as seriously as . . . White females do in health care. That's just like how it is, unfortunately. So, I feel like being an advocate for yourself is important. And letting them know about how you're treated and just like keep speaking up about it until something is done . . . don't let them treat you poorly . . . don't allow it. Always be an advocate for yourself. (*Asia, mid-20s, cisgender woman*)

Similarly, transgender and nonbinary individuals also encounter cultural incompetence from providers in health care that can contribute to health disparities. A 2018 study of reproductive health care needs in individuals assigned female at birth revealed challenges for LGBTQ individuals including the assumptions that fertility is sought and all individuals seeking health care identify as women (as evidenced by "women's health" in clinic titles), as well as direct discrimination from providers (Wingo et al., 2018). Gender-based bias stems from cisgender and gender binary assumptions that remain prominent in society, such as that transitioning involves moving from one binary gender to the other via surgical procedures (Austin & Goodman, 2018). Given that nonbinary individuals may not experience gender as binary and therefore do not transition in the traditional sense, assumptions that they do may explain why nonbinary individuals report more misgendering and negative experiences with health care providers than binary individuals (Goldberg et al., 2019). Providers may be unaware that the currently accepted model of transgender health is not bound by binary gender or that distress is often grounded in stigma rather than diverse gender identity itself (Bockting, 2009).

Individuals I interviewed experienced gender-based cultural incompetence in health care surrounding the assumption that all PCOS patients are straight, cisgender women. This assumption can be distressing for individuals with diverse gender identities and often is accompanied by the additional expectation that all individuals with PCOS want treatment to feminize the masculinizing symptoms of PCOS. Because they may identify outside of womanhood, they may find aesthetic appeal in the masculinizing symptoms of PCOS and experience confusion about what treatment they actually need for their health beyond ones that change their appearance, as illustrated by Jo:

> I had a lot of difficult experiences with doctors . . . it's hard to gear myself up to go to the doctor. . . . I'm going to be asked if I want to get pregnant and then be told I'm a great candidate for electrolysis and . . . be offered birth control and . . . have all these assumptions made about me. . . . Most of the things that people think about . . . don't . . . apply to me because I have been privileged and I'm not interested in pregnancy and I'm not interested in heterosexuality or femininity. . . . I think the . . . social understanding and the medical understanding of the condition is very much based on . . . fertility within . . . heterosexual monogamous context. . . . And so, that can be very alienating to people who are not part of that, who either want to have children outside of that . . . heterosexual context . . . and also to people who are just not interested in having biological children. . . . I think that's very invalidating to anyone who doesn't want to have children and has the condition . . . and especially, to queer people . . . there's this idea of compulsory heterosexuality, and if you've dropped out of that and you're not like bestowing your supposed biological purpose. I think that's kind of . . . stigmatized, and doctors can contribute to that. . . . I also think the . . . idea of how you need to treat certain symptoms with PCOS for purely aesthetic reasons is very much based on this notion

of what a desirable woman is like. That's . . . sold to us through a variety of means and is very much based on like White male gaze. And so, I guess in some ways, . . . being somebody who's not part of that system, . . . not trying to look a certain way to be . . . desirable to a heterosexual man, I think it's less pressure in some way because you don't have to do that. But it's also . . . everything you're being told about what the condition means and how you can or should treat it and what your options are and what the assumptions are, I think that's . . . invalidating a lot of times or confusing or frustrating or unhelpful to queer and trans people, especially . . . for me and other people I know who are transmasculine and . . . having facial and body hair is super affirming to us . . . going to the doctor and being offered testosterone blockers and birth control and different types of hair removal procedures . . . it's frustrating and invalidating. (*Jo, late 20s, genderqueer/nonbinary*)

Some described a blatant omission of transgender-affirming health care (Rory's excerpt) or negative treatment from providers they attributed to gender identity (Aiden's excerpt).

There's just . . . none—trans comprehensive health care in general. . . . So for people who are trans and have PCOS, there's nothing at all. Double whammy . . . to be able to bridge those experiences, and . . . be comprehensive of those experiences, . . . health care professionals generally aren't. (*Rory, early 20s, nonbinary*)

I also initiated a conversation about . . . identifying as trans. . . . I was asking . . . "Could you give any more information about how something like HRT might affect me having PCOS with insulin resistance and the already elevated testosterone levels?" And then I said, . . . "Would you be able to help me sort . . . that out, or do you have any recommendations for an endocrinologist or someone who specializes in this type of thing?" And instead of giving me . . . unbiased, objective information, she decided to use . . . a scare tactic. She said that she had a patient that also identified as trans and . . . this particular person transitioned so quickly that now they were . . . unrecognizable as a female. And she was . . . warning me about this and said that this patient . . . deeply regretted their transition, and so . . . I should think very carefully and perhaps not even consider that at all. . . . I was hoping . . . she would provide . . . information that was . . . unbiased and objective . . . but instead, she chose to . . . put this other patient on blast, and I don't even know if she had permission from that person, or if that person . . . even really existed . . . maybe she made it up entirely. I don't know, but it was just a very negative experience. And I didn't go back to her, certainly. And it took me about a year to sort of work up the courage to find a new provider. (*Aiden, mid-20s, transmasculine*)

These encounters reflect lack of knowledge among providers about gender diversity and health care needs. Marsh's provider argued in favor of medications to reduce testosterone, citing the negative impact that high testosterone would have on health. Marsh perceived this as pressure to normalize to a more feminine body. Marsh returned to the provider after self-identifying their gender as nonbinary. This time, the provider offered to take the PCOS diagnosis off their medical chart, citing that Marsh was now a man. In actuality, Marsh did *not* identify as a man (the provider misgendered the patient), and they still had ovaries (the provider misunderstood the needs of a nonbinary patient with PCOS):

> Everyone assumes that you're a girl and that you want . . . to be normal . . . you want to be normalized . . . including . . . a doctor I still see. . . . I was seeing him just a couple of years ago, . . . he did a blood test and said, "Your testosterone is high for a woman and I'm going to put you on spironolactone." And I said, ". . . I have a partner who's a trans woman who's on that as a testosterone blocker . . . doesn't that make you pee a lot and have a lot of other side effects like brain fog . . . and what's the problem with having high testosterone? It gives me high sex drive. It makes me feel good . . . maybe it makes me grow some body hair, but . . . I don't have a problem with my body hair. So why would I be on that?" And he was . . . telling me that having high testosterone was a health problem that could cause me to have . . . high blood pressure and heart attacks . . . he wrote down that I refused the medication. And then . . . I came out as nonbinary and started taking testosterone. . . . And when I came back to him [provider], he suddenly changed his tune and was like, "Okay, this is fine." And it was like . . . high testosterone was gonna kill me, but now it's fine? So, there's just all this . . . pressure to normalize you and . . . normalize your body. And the things that your body is doing naturally are . . . wrong and bad. . . . More recently, he said that he could take that [PCOS] off of my chart because I'm a man now, which I am not. I don't identify as a man. I also still have all my ovaries and I have not had a hysterectomy. . . . He said that he could take it off my chart now because I'm on testosterone, which . . . doesn't make any sense . . . just because I'm on testosterone. (*Marsh, mid-30s, nonbinary*)

Similarly, Charlie's excerpt summarizes such challenges of finding gender-affirming medical care in the context of PCOS when treatment recommendations are based in a gender binary and feminization. As evidenced by Charlie's frustration about gender diverse individuals always needing to seek out their own options for care, the excerpt also shows a need for improved communication from providers for why certain treatments are being offered.

> And just the immediate reaction from doctors is, "Now that we know you have PCOS . . . these are the treatments that you have." And it's just an immediate push [to] get rid of facial hair. . . . The push to go back on . . . birth control was pretty strong. . . . And I really couldn't understand what exactly was . . . the need, because . . . I know a lot of trans men, that . . . don't have their period continuously. . . . And I think I got an explanation [of] why, essentially because it sounds like trans men . . . with taking testosterone, they get to a threshold of not adding to the uterine lining. And . . . then . . . it's not an issue. But most people don't even know that. . . . I was only able to get that explanation whenever I . . . went to a doctor who . . . has done a lot of work with trans people . . . they basically have a trans clinic. . . . But that kind of explanation,

I was not getting from my previous OBGYN or from my general practitioner. . . . It's very standardized with "this is what's recommended because this is how we understand it." . . . And the alternative isn't even . . . offering testosterone . . . unless, of course, you're specifically . . . asking for that . . . the standardized health care is based on a binary system, essentially. . . . And if I hadn't had to go out of my way to talk to other trans people who have PCOS and like what they've experienced . . . that's definitely . . . frustrating. . . . Trans people have had to take care of their own medical health care for quite some time. (*Charlie, late 20s, genderfluid*)

Cultural incompetence in health care may lead individuals with PCOS to avoid health care altogether or not adhere to recommended treatments. Limited research has examined treatment adherence in individuals with PCOS (Parker et al., 2020). We know from social psychological research on intergroup relations that patients of stigmatized groups harbor prejudice concerns and mistrust of providers, whereas trust and satisfaction contribute to medical adherence (Major et al., 2013). Analysis of the 2015 U.S. transgender survey that captured more than 20,000 transgender, gender nonconforming, and nonbinary individuals across the country revealed that nearly a quarter of trans individuals avoided seeking health care out of fear of being mistreated within the health care system (Lerner et al., 2021). Among the experiences that predicted greater avoidance of the system included verbal harassment, having to educate providers about trans issues, invasive questioning, and being refused care. Indeed, discrimination in health care can keep LGBT individuals from effective treatments for chronic illnesses (Jowett & Peel, 2009).

What About Satisfaction?

To be fair, not all health care encounters are negative. In fact, half of the individuals with PCOS whom I interviewed did report some positive aspect to their health care encounters. In some instances, both positive and negative behaviors were exhibited in exchanges with the same provider. Whereas the bottom line with PCOS health care seems to be that it leaves a lot to be desired, the reports of positive health care encounters may shed light on what is working and how other experiences might be improved for patients with PCOS. As shown in this section, the positive aspects of health care tend to reflect the opposite of the negative: collaboration on the best treatment options rather than assumptions, affirmation of identity rather than bias, and understanding about PCOS rather than lack of knowledge.

Collaboration may be one key to positive health care experiences with PCOS. This collaboration may best surround provision of options for treatment rather than a one-size-fits-all approach. Kim, for instance, described being more satisfied with providers who were collaborative in nature and not solely focused on medications for treating all the PCOS symptoms:

> At the moment, I feel pretty good because I feel like I have providers who are really supportive and make decisions with me rather than for me. I would say that hasn't always been the case . . . I've had a lot of providers who haven't been really supportive or collaborative. . . . It took me a long [time] to find folks that I felt like were collaborative providers and weren't just trying to give me pharma [medication] to get me to go away . . . they'd sit and talk with me about a plan or how I wanted to manage or where I was comfortable. . . . So, at the moment, I would say I feel pretty satisfied with my medical management team. (*Kim, mid-30s, cisgender woman*)

Kim further clarified that not everyone wants all symptoms treated. For some, facial and body hair are not distressing and may even be gender affirming. Therefore, providers should know that treatments to reduce hyperandrogenism in PCOS may not be relevant for all their patients with PCOS. Treating PCOS may conflict with gender identity.

> I would want collaboration from a care provider . . . for me, I wouldn't just want "here are the symptoms that you have, here's how we normally treat them. So we're just going to do that . . ." I don't necessarily want to manage all my symptoms medically. As I mentioned, I don't . . . take anything for having excess facial hair or . . . hair loss on top of my head. . . . that didn't fit for me. . . . I want a collaborative care provider who could talk about different options for different things, for different symptoms. There isn't one set . . . regimen for care. (*Kim, mid-30s, cisgender woman*)

Not surprisingly, positive health care encounters for PCOS involved providers who were educated about PCOS. Individuals further specified that the knowledgeable providers often specialized in PCOS. Moreover, encounters with knowledgeable and affirming providers appeared to be life changing for patients with PCOS. Excerpts by Jack and Amethyst illustrate.

> I thankfully have a great doctor. . . . PCOS [is] part of her focus. And she was the one who—who did everything and figured out that's what I've been dealing with my whole life . . . the more recent experiences that I've had, specifically the last two doctors were . . . honestly life changing. (*Jack, mid-30s, nonbinary*)

> Whenever I moved out to [bigger city] . . . there's a lot more doctors who have different studies here, so I was able to find a specialist . . . once I got a specialist . . . I was able to find someone who solely studied PCOS . . . it definitely helped me a lot more and I was definitely a lot more happy with my experience. (*Amethyst, mid-20s, cisgender woman*)

Health care encounters also were positive when they were identity affirming, such as when providers used appropriate names and pronouns, as illustrated by Aiden's narrative. An approach that reflected beliefs that individuals could be healthy at any body size rather than one focused solely on weight loss made a difference. With this philosophy, individuals with PCOS could approach their bodies and health more positively, as illustrated by Dylan's narrative. These types of positive encounters in health care often involved alternative practitioners such as acupuncturists, physical therapists, and midwives rather than traditional health care providers.

> I was able to find someone that has been really wonderful and that's taken really good care of me. The experiences that I had between the two are like night and day. My new provider . . . took the time to listen and is . . . very understanding and uses my name and my pronouns like I've asked. And it just makes me feel comfortable and hasn't even dared to say anything even close to what the previous provider has. And she always talks very . . . carefully and . . . spells things out and just gives me time to make an informed decision regarding my health. . . . So, it's been a much more positive experience with my new provider . . . she . . . tried to dig deeper into how . . . hormones are playing a role. And since I've had the . . . implant . . . progesterone only, not the estrogen . . . that has really helped with . . . symptoms . . . as far as the pain, for long periods. I haven't had much pain since that point . . . my period has pretty much stopped altogether. . . . It's been really important to . . . take . . . a multifaceted approach, and this is a doctor that I feel like I really can talk to. . . . Sometimes it just takes someone who is willing to really dig deep and work with you . . . and not just . . . assume and just prescribe something. (*Aiden, mid-20s, transmasculine*)

> Physicians that I have had experiences with that have been really well versed in this and really supportive of me have all had a health-at-every-size framework around how they navigate bodies in general, which gives me a lot . . . more room to think about the care of my body rather than the punishment and shrinking of my body. . . . It was from that lens that I was able to . . . think about my food as a source of fuel, and . . . how I want to navigate energy rather than like what would make me fat or not, which was the framework I was given previously. So that . . . really enabled me to think more holistically about my health. And it's enabled me to . . . embrace movement in a way that wasn't punishment. And . . . both psychologically and . . . in the health of my body . . . that framework and model has really increased my health. (*Dylan, late 20s, genderqueer*)

CONCLUSION

Many individuals living with PCOS are consistently dissatisfied with their health care experiences because their providers lack knowledge about PCOS, resulting in delayed diagnosis. Poor provider–patient interactions (which reflect dismissiveness, weight bias, and cultural incompetence) additionally create a context of inadequate PCOS health care resources. Meanwhile, individuals living with PCOS are at increased risk for major chronic diseases that likely mean they are accessing the health care system even more frequently over time. Evidence presented here from individuals living with PCOS whom I interviewed, combined with the existing scientific literature on health care encounters, underscores the need for change in PCOS health care in the United States. Change should focus on increasing provider knowledge about PCOS, sensitivity about stigma and bias, and collaboration with patients about treatment options. Because similarly negative health care encounters of individuals with PCOS have been reported in other countries, presumably these changes could be implemented globally to better address PCOS. In the next chapter, I call for positive changes to address these shortcomings in PCOS health care. Moreover, using the findings of this book as a whole, I lay the foundation for building a psychological science of PCOS.

7

A PCOS CALL TO ACTION

Interventions, Advocacy, and Psychological Science

No action without research, no research without action.

–Kurt Lewin (Marrow, 1969, p. 163)

Something I often do in my writing is to bring the story full circle—to strike at the end an echo of a note that was sounded at the beginning. It gratifies my sense of symmetry, and it also pleases the reader, completing with its resonance the journey we set out on together.

–William Zinsser (2013, p. 65), On Writing Well

The preceding six chapters have addressed myriad psychosocial experiences reported by individuals living with polycystic ovary syndrome (PCOS). In this book, I have introduced PCOS and its symptoms, along with the silence surrounding the syndrome (Chapter 1), argued that PCOS symptoms can be stigmatizing (Chapter 2), explored the gendered embodiment of PCOS (Chapter 3), described social support and close relationship processes in PCOS context (Chapter 4), uncovered both psychological symptoms and the growth possible in the lives of individuals living with PCOS (Chapter 5), and

https://doi.org/10.1037/0000337-008

examined the inadequate PCOS health care resources combined with health risks of the syndrome (Chapter 6). This final chapter summarizes and translates the psychosocial experiences this book underscored into three main areas of future PCOS work: interventions, advocacy, and psychological science. The road map for future work uses an ecological systems framework to approach this future work at multiple levels to move forward the ultimate goal of this book, which is to replace the problem of invisibility or silence around the syndrome with science, building a psychology of PCOS and improving the lives of individuals living with it.

TRANSLATING WHAT WE HAVE LEARNED TO INTERVENTIONS

Before considering specific action steps, let us pause and reflect on the very real psychosocial challenges that individuals living with PCOS face daily that were summarized in this book. Given the multiple psychosocial implications of the condition, individuals living with PCOS potentially encounter enacted and internalized stigma, threats to gender identity and body image, challenges in close relationships, psychological symptoms, and risk for major chronic health problems in a context of severely inadequate health care resources—simultaneously. Further, because of the invisibility and stigma associated with PCOS, many appear to suffer in silence. At the same time, some are negotiating PCOS daily in a journey toward self-acceptance and positive personal growth. Some even view PCOS symptoms as aligned with their diverse gender identities.

These revelations need to be translated into a path forward that reduces psychosocial risk and enhances growth and quality of life in individuals living with PCOS. One path forward presumably should involve mental health care. Given psychologists' expertise, they would be ideal professionals to facilitate reduced psychosocial risk and enhanced positive growth. Regarding mental health care, however, it is unclear whether individuals with PCOS seek psychotherapy for PCOS symptoms specifically or whether therapists know about PCOS. Individuals I interviewed varied in terms of whether they had received mental health treatment, as well as whether they talked directly about PCOS diagnosis or symptoms with their mental health provider. Many who sought treatment, such as Kendall (*early 20s, nonbinary*), described it as helpful to them as they managed their PCOS and related psychological symptoms: "I just learned through just talk therapy how to really just build my self-esteem and just love myself for once and just love the body I'm in."

Admittedly, though, mental health providers varied in how knowledgeable they were about PCOS and how to be helpful to their clients with PCOS. These conflicting reports of both helpfulness and needing to educate their providers to be most helpful were voiced by Jordan:

> I was in a fat therapy group for a couple of years. . . . Everyone in the group had PCOS . . . we would end up talking [about PCOS] a lot. And that was really helpful, especially to be able to process that with a therapist. I just try to be kinder to myself when I know that the things that I'm dealing with in my body are because of the PCOS. Just a lot of . . . positive self-talk, things like that. (*Jordan, late 20s, nonbinary/agender/sometimes woman*)

> I didn't start going to therapy because of my issues because of PCOS. But it is something that I do talk about with my therapist who I've been seeing for about 3 years now. And it is something that I've talked to with my last couple of psychiatrists as we tried to figure out . . . what medications would work for me and my mental health issues. . . . My therapist has been great, but I found that I had to educate them about what PCOS was and how it would affect me. My psychiatrist—I've never had one that really seemed to get it. Where again . . . I have to educate them on what my symptoms were and what kind of treatment I might need from them. (*Jordan, late 20s, nonbinary/agender/ sometimes woman*)

Thus, I begin this call to action by suggesting ways to improve available mental health care resources before moving to suggested improvements in health care more broadly. I focus on the need for continuing education for mental health providers and interventions targeting psychosocial impacts of PCOS that improve mental health and care.

Clinical Interventions to Address Psychological Risk and Growth in PCOS

The chapters in this book highlight the need for interventions to reduce negative psychosocial impacts of PCOS symptoms and to facilitate psychological growth in individuals living with PCOS. Limited psychological intervention work has specifically focused on individuals with PCOS. A go-to treatment for individuals with PCOS is lifestyle modification, including diet and exercise (Teede et al., 2018). As this book has shown, individuals living with PCOS may perceive this go-to treatment from health care providers as weight bias. Further, whereas exercise can improve insulin resistance, more research is needed to determine effectiveness in improving mental health in PCOS (Conte et al., 2015). Reframing exercise interventions to improve mental health rather than weight loss could result in more positive reception from patients as well. Additionally, interventions aimed directly at unhealthy cognitions might be more helpful avenues to improving psychological outcomes in those living with PCOS. I provide a couple of intervention options that might prove fruitful in addressing psychological growth and positive outcomes in PCOS. As well, a couple of individuals I interviewed shared that resisting the dominant culture's body shaming through body positivity approaches has made a positive impact on their self-acceptance (see Appendix B for suggested reading).

Cognitive behavior therapy (CBT) techniques address negative thought patterns that contribute to negative mood or problematic behavior and might prove helpful for PCOS. For example, acceptance and commitment therapy (ACT) may be particularly relevant for PCOS given its focus on psychological flexibility and acceptance, aligning behaviors with values. Indeed, ACT has been shown to be effective in improving body image and self-esteem immediately and 1 month after intervention in individuals with PCOS compared with controls (Moradi et al., 2020). Two other recent intervention studies have shown that CBT can increase quality of life in women with PCOS. One of these, a U.S.-based study, examined a general lifestyle intervention plus CBT condition against a general lifestyle-intervention-only condition over 16 weeks and found greater quality of life and less depression when CBT was included (Cooney et al., 2018). The other, an Iran-based study, compared an 8-week CBT intervention with a no-intervention control and found greater quality of life with CBT (Abdollahi et al., 2019).

Additional therapeutic techniques may confer improvements in psychological outcomes for individuals with PCOS but need to be examined within this population. Self-compassion comprising mindfulness, self-kindness, and recognition of the common humanity in one's suffering (Neff, 2003) may be a fruitful avenue for intervention, particularly because it is essentially antithetical to shame and stigma (S. L. Williams et al., 2021). Although not yet examined in individuals with PCOS, self-compassion interventions may have salutary effects on psychological outcomes of PCOS given its benefits for body dissatisfaction and thereby reduced distress (Rahimi-Ardabili et al., 2018). Indeed, a self-compassion intervention reduced internalized weight stigma and improved body satisfaction from pre-intervention to 3-month post-intervention (Forbes et al., 2020). As well, the mindfulness aspect of self-compassion has been shown to reduce depression and anxiety and improve quality of life in individuals with PCOS in Greece who completed an 8-week mindfulness-only intervention compared with the control condition (Stefanaki et al., 2015). Clinicians may find that increased self-compassion may naturally help move individuals with PCOS from shame to acceptance of their bodies. Future research should explore this possibility.

Therapists would benefit from knowing about the psychosocial impacts of PCOS and subsequently tailoring therapeutic interventions to the symptoms of PCOS with which individuals are dealing. As shown in this book, PCOS is experienced differently based on the compilation of symptoms individuals report and individual factors such as gender identity. For some, body image and weight stigma can have a considerable impact on mental health. Future intervention work in individuals with PCOS might target internalized weight stigma and body satisfaction. For others, the most impactful symptom may be infertility. Because individual-, couple-, and external-level factors interact to produce the impact of infertility, future intervention work should consider these complex interrelations (Ridenour et al., 2009). Moreover, therapists should also demonstrate cultural competence, considering context and inter-sectionality in their work with clients. The American Psychological Associ-ation has several sets of guidelines that may assist clinicians in their work with clients with diverse sexual, gender, and racial/ethnic groups (https://www.apa.org/about/policy/approved-guidelines). Across diverse groups, these guidelines cover important therapeutic considerations such as unconscious bias, minority stress, and intersectionality. Clinicians might consider minority stress interventions when working with diverse groups with PCOS (Chaudoir et al., 2017).

Interventions to Improve PCOS Health Care

Another path toward improving quality of life in individuals living with PCOS involves addressing the inadequate PCOS-specific health care resources, described in Chapter 6. As a social psychologist, I certainly hold no direct knowledge of health care and what it is like to be a health care provider. Furthermore, my understanding of health care is limited to the U.S. health care system—where I live and where the individuals I interviewed live. Thus, I focus on the areas in which psychological science can offer help via theories and frameworks to help improve provider knowledge and interactions with patients. Social, health, and clinical psychologists in particular may ideally offer ways to improve the health care experience, given the integration of clinical psychology into primary health care and the relevant translational science in these areas.

Further, although I do not deny the very real structural limitations placed on providers by the health care system itself, the suggestions that follow focus on the psychological contributions within the areas of health care presented as most important for individuals living with PCOS. This approach centers on the lived experiences that people with PCOS have had with the health care system. The bottom line is that health care *must* change. It is unfathomable that in the 21st century we are still grappling with diagnosis and treatment for PCOS. After more than 85 years since PCOS was formally identified, doctors still lack knowledge of the syndrome. Combine that reality with the continued lack of cultural sensitivity of providers toward their patients and we have a recipe for continued delays in diagnosis, biased interactions, and increased risk of worse health outcomes. By addressing these areas of health care, presumably the patient experience and time to diagnosis of PCOS will improve.

Increasing Provider Knowledge About PCOS

Given the consistency of the reports by individuals living with PCOS, the most obvious change needed in health care is improved knowledge about PCOS among their providers. Increased knowledge about signs and symptoms of the syndrome in providers would presumably reduce the delays experienced before obtaining a PCOS diagnosis (Gibson-Helm et al., 2018b). Provider knowledge would increase patient satisfaction with provider interactions as well. It seems that primary care physicians in particular may lack appropriate and sufficient education about PCOS (Gibson-Helm et al., 2014). Patients can perceive this deficiency as less trust in the provider's ability to treat PCOS (whereas they do not harbor a lack of trust in provider ability to treat general health; Lin et al., 2018). This is particularly unfortunate because primary care physicians are typically the first step for individuals seeking diagnosis (Sills et al., 2001). Efforts to improve the knowledge of health care providers are clearly needed, but the pathway to increased knowledge is less clear. A survey of nearly 1,500 health care providers in multiple countries revealed that multiple methods of education (education materials, workshops, website, email) may reach the most providers, and these educational activities should be codeveloped with providers to gain buy-in and address any barriers to knowledge uptake (Gibson-Helm et al., 2018a). Professional societies may be well positioned to create resources or learning opportunities (Gibson-Helm et al., 2018b).

Another area of needed change in health care involves mental health. Because individuals with PCOS often have comorbid mental health concerns, such as depression, anxiety, quality of life, and eating disorders, PCOS experts emphasize the need for health care providers to screen for depression, anxiety, and eating disorders at the time they are diagnosing PCOS (Dokras et al., 2018). Yet a systematic review of 35 published papers on patients' and providers' health care needs and experiences of receiving or providing care regarding PCOS revealed that psychological correlates of

PCOS are less recognized by providers and that patients value this particular knowledge among physicians (Gibson-Helm et al., 2018b). The authors of the review paper recommended that education material about PCOS consist of biopsychosocial information and that such a resource be developed collaboratively by patients and providers. Others have suggested that providers ask patients to complete a measure on quality of life to understand more fully how the syndrome affects them (Crete & Adamshick, 2011), which would allow for a more holistic picture of their health rather than an individual symptom approach. One solution to this problem of recognition of PCOS diagnosis and corresponding psychological outcomes is an integrated care approach. For instance, comprehensive care offered through a center that involves multiple disciplines communicating with one another could at once address medical, social, psychological, and other burdens of PCOS (Dokras & Witchel, 2014). Another strategy would be to integrate behavioral health into primary care to ensure the social and psychological aspects of PCOS experience become regularly addressed in health care. With integrated care, medical and behavioral health work together as a team to carry out treatment plans involving both medical and behavioral components and treat the whole person, which is particularly effective for managing chronic conditions (Rajesh et al., 2019).

Addressing Weight Stigma in PCOS Health Care
Individuals living with PCOS consistently report that health care providers focus solely on their weight and weight loss during health care visits. Indeed, individuals report frustration, shame, and anger about physicians' continued suggestion that they lose weight without acknowledgment that PCOS is not caused by their weight—in fact, lean patients have PCOS too, losing weight does not cure PCOS, and it is incredibly difficult to lose weight due to PCOS. Because being overweight is a stigmatized condition itself, PCOS patients perceive providers' focus on weight as blame for their weight and for their PCOS.

Providers' focus on weight during PCOS health care visits may at least partially be explained by the fact that the 2018 international guidelines for treating PCOS focuses on lifestyle management by way of weight loss or diet and exercise (Teede et al., 2018). Thus, it may even be expected that providers would discuss weight in conjunction with patients as a PCOS management strategy. A specific challenge of offering a medicalized treatment regimen consisting of exercise and other lifestyle modifications through diet may imply to the patient with PCOS that it is the lack of healthy lifestyle behaviors that led to their condition (Woodward et al., 2020).

Yet although interactions between patients and providers regarding weight may be further complicated by the view of some providers that PCOS is caused by lifestyle behaviors, a definitive cause of PCOS is unknown. One published paper referenced PCOS as a lifestyle disorder along with Type 2 diabetes and gestational diabetes (Kozica et al., 2012). In this work, the authors stated that insulin resistance undergirds these lifestyle conditions, which is precipitated by obesity and high caloric diets combined with inactivity. Whereas some research shows that those with PCOS display more negative health behaviors than those with other "lifestyle disorders" (Kozica et al., 2012), importantly, other research finds no differences between those with and without PCOS in diet suggestive of obesity driving PCOS development (Azziz, 2016). Weight is not the cause of PCOS, individuals did not cause their own PCOS, and, therefore, weight loss does not cure PCOS. There is no cure for PCOS.

Because of the reality that PCOS symptoms such as weight are stigmatizing, providers must be aware of and address the weight bias and shame perceived by individuals with PCOS seeking care from them. In addition to the suggestions related to weight management, the 2018 international guidelines for PCOS treatment also suggested that providers consider the stigma attached to weight when talking with PCOS patients (Teede et al., 2018). Future interventions should educate providers on ways they could discuss stigma directly with their patients. Psychologists with expertise in stigma and health may be best suited to provide suggestions on ways to communicate with patients about weight-based stigma while explaining that the suggested management strategies involving diet and exercise stem from a set of guidelines developed by international experts in PCOS. By recognizing the stigmatizing nature of a weight-centric approach, providers may become more open to alternative or nondiet approaches that are also effective for healthy living (Clifford et al., 2015). These less stigmatizing options promote healthful behavior change while respecting body shape and size. One specific example, *Health at Every Size* (Association for Size Diversity and Health, n.d.), an approach that emphasizes health equity, inclusivity for all body sizes and shapes, and ending weight bias by recognizing that healthy and unhealthy people can exist at all sizes, was recommended as a positive alternative by individuals I interviewed. Some evidence suggests that this approach can be efficacious in improving some metabolic indicators (Bacon et al., 2005) and body acceptance (O'Hara et al., 2021).

Addressing the stigma in the exam room seems paramount especially given that weight bias exists more broadly in health care (as I described in Chapter 6) and has implications for patient health. Unfortunately, a systematic review of interventions designed to reduce weight bias in health professionals showed a lack of rigorous and efficacious interventions to reduce weight bias in health care (Alberga et al., 2016). This may be an additional area where psychologists with expertise in weight stigma and intervention work could assist in improving provider interactions with patients. In this regard, researchers Melissa Himelein and Samuel Thatcher (2006a) suggested that physicians be cautious when suggesting weight loss to individuals with PCOS without providing support for body dissatisfaction they might be experiencing. Given the potential risk for eating disorders, health care providers must use greater care in communicating with patients about reasons for lifestyle recommendations and offer further support such as referrals to psychologists. This shift in approach would require more awareness and understanding from physicians about the likely reciprocal relations among body dissatisfaction, depression, dieting, and weight.

Increasing Provider Cultural Competence

Culturally competent health care is essential to improving patient satisfaction (Govere & Govere, 2016). Individuals with PCOS whom I interviewed offered suggestions on what could improve PCOS health care that were reflective of cultural competence: (a) not making assumptions about a PCOS patient's gender, sexuality, or desire to conceive children; (b) awareness of identity-related challenges due to limited PCOS treatment options that center on aesthetic qualities of the condition that some might not want to change; and (c) more understanding of trans and nonbinary gender health care needs. These are illustrated by Jo and Rory's excerpts:

> I think an important thing would be to not assume that everyone who has it [PCOS] is a woman. Not everyone who has it is heterosexual. Not everyone who has it wants to have children. . . . And, I think . . . not only asking people what symptoms they are having, but . . . what symptoms are bothering them is important. Rather than assuming that . . . what bothers some people will bother everyone and needs to be treated, especially if it's basically an aesthetic thing. And, I think that . . . telling people what all of their options are rather than just being like, "Well, we'll put you on birth control" because not everybody wants that. And it can be kind of coercive to tell people that their only option is to have these . . . specific hormones in their body if that's not their body's natural state. And that's not going to result in what they want. (*Jo, late 20s, genderqueer/nonbinary*)

> I'm really wary of the ways in which . . . doctors use their authority. And also, some people come in to . . . get help and before they diagnose you, they shame the symptoms they might be having. And then the way they use their authority in order to shame people. And I think I've been through that a lot . . . the center

of . . . my experience and . . . things I think need to change . . . comes from . . . the shaming that comes with the diagnosis. . . . I wish there was . . . a culture that was more . . . trans inclusive and . . . able to question . . . this very . . . binary understanding of gender. (*Rory, early 20s, nonbinary*)

Increasing culturally competent PCOS health care for individuals who are gender diverse might best be achieved by combining general improvements within the practice with specific considerations for how gender intersects with PCOS experience. In general, providers could improve gender inclusiveness of their practices in small ways such as by learning LGBTQ terminology, representing diverse gender and pronouns on intake paperwork, and diversifying the literature and photographs in the waiting room (Kattari et al., 2020). However, these surface-level indicators of a welcoming practice alone are insufficient and should be combined with deeper inclusive practices that would likely require more education, such as through the National LGBTQIA+ Health Education Center, which is part of the Fenway Institute and provides programming and consultation to health care organizations to promote quality health care in their gender diverse patient population (https://www.lgbtqiahealtheducation.org/). More specific to the PCOS experience, providers should be aware that PCOS is not a condition occurring in women but rather in individuals assigned female at birth (or those born with ovaries). Avoiding woman-centric language in relation to PCOS and instead using gender-neutral language is key to evidencing awareness of this fact. Moreover, because not everyone with PCOS is a woman, at least some gender diverse clients may not want to treat their PCOS if it means feminizing their physical characteristics. Of course, one of the resulting challenges of gender awareness is the uncertainty of how to treat PCOS to prevent the long-term health problems of PCOS while still respecting a patient's gender identity.

Culturally competent care should also involve the racial/ethnic identity of individuals of all genders living with PCOS. Culturally competent care for individuals of various racial and ethnic groups is increasingly required by state government and medical organizations (Govere & Govere, 2016). For instance, graduate accrediting bodies call for education surrounding health disparities in medical training. Recall that health disparities are those systematic differences in health outcomes that minoritized groups experience relative to majority groups. These disparities are attributable to the identity-specific oppression and related stress they encounter. Despite this call, graduate medical education curriculum falls short of this goal, and program directors have identified barriers to a health disparities curriculum that are reflective of lack of time and faculty and institutional support for it (Dupras et al., 2020).

Didactic training on health disparities may not provide the depth of focus on racism as the cause of health inequities as do educational programs developed to address racism directly (White-Davis et al., 2018). Didactic and interactive learning opportunities that directly address racism in health care (White-Davis et al., 2018) must be tested and translated to improve patient care.

Training specifically aimed at improving cultural competence has been shown to increase competence in healthcare providers and improve patient satisfaction (Govere & Govere, 2016). However, primarily didactic training in health disparities may not provide the skills needed to demonstrate cultural humility (Dupras et al., 2020). Cultural humility rather than competence may be needed to promote the sensitivity needed in providers to transform patient care. Whereas cultural competence implies there is an endpoint of the learning process when one can reach expert knowledge about diverse groups, cultural humility is a continual process of learning and self-reflection (Buchanan et al., 2020). Going a step further, an intersectional approach to cultural humility may best center the experiences of individuals with marginalized identities and the oppressions that undergird differences in life outcomes (Buchanan et al., 2020). In regard to health care, an intersectional cultural humility approach would require continual reflection on one's biases, recognition of the impact of systemic oppression, life-long learning, and acknowledgment that mistakes might be made and that one may never achieve mastery (Buchanan et al., 2020). A provider using an approach based in intersectional cultural humility would likely hold fewer assumptions based on stereotypes about groups and more consideration of the individual person in context.

A trauma-informed approach to PCOS health care also may improve PCOS-related health care experiences. I offer this approach not because PCOS has a direct link to trauma but because individuals with PCOS—especially those from marginalized groups—may experience intrapersonal, interpersonal, and structural trauma due to stigma and unfair treatment, including within the health care system (Boudreau et al., 2021). The principles of trauma-informed care promote a welcoming environment in which patients feel safe and respected. These six principles are (a) safety; (b) trustworthiness and transparency; (c) peer support from others with similar experiences; (d) collaboration and mutuality; (e) empowerment, voice, and choice; and (f) cultural, historical, and gender issues related to moving past biases (Substance Abuse and Mental Health Services Administration, 2014). With these principles, a trauma-informed approach to health care acknowledges past trauma and minimizes additional trauma (Poteat & Singh, 2017). Trust in one's provider and receipt of safe, transparent, and collaborative care may not only prevent additional trauma but also promote resilience (Poteat & Singh, 2017). Small changes to provider communication and understanding implemented universally regardless of patients' past trauma history can improve patient-centeredness of care and reflect awareness of trauma's effects (Raja et al., 2015).

ADVOCACY

Because this book has underscored the silence and invisibility of PCOS in society and in psychological science, any call to action must include advocacy. Who should advocate for PCOS? Most certainly one answer to that question includes organizations whose sole mission is to improve the lives of individuals with PCOS, which is a current source of incredible advocacy work being done. One specific organization I became familiar with when I began this book project is PCOS Challenge: The National Polycystic Ovary Syndrome Association, which has more than 55,000 PCOS patients as members and is growing. The leaders and many volunteers of this advocacy and patient support organization seek to raise awareness about PCOS and reduce risk of disease. They carry out their mission through large-scale awareness campaigns, direct advocacy work with Congress, connection with national agencies that fund research, and an annual symposium featuring leaders in PCOS research and patient panels, among many other activities. A recent result of their important advocacy work was a workshop hosted by the National Institutes of Health in October 2021, focused on identifying future research priorities in cardiovascular risk in PCOS. Thus, advocacy organizations that exist in the United States and internationally can promote large-scale change by encouraging collaboration among providers, researchers, patients, and policy makers.

Considering other sources of advocacy work, researchers also are ideal advocates. During my own professional training as a psychological scientist, I did not directly learn advocacy skills. However, researchers can be ideal advocates for important social and health issues like PCOS. The American Psychological Association and its specialty divisions list advocacy as part of their charge. These organizations pride themselves on having access to experts holding scientific knowledge in particular societal issues that can influence policy and helping scientists translate their research into action (see https://www.apaservices.org/advocacy/get-involved).

Finally, individuals living with PCOS can use their own voices, sharing their PCOS experiences to increase visibility and break the silence. Using our own platforms with friends and family or even social media can have an impact within the immediate community. Individual voices can be further elevated when patients partner with advocacy organizations. For instance, each year PCOS Challenge organizes an advocacy day during which patients, researchers, and health care providers come together to talk with politicians. Patients share their own PCOS stories to highlight their lived experiences to provide the emotional connection to PCOS that representatives of the government would not otherwise have. This grassroots advocacy can affect change at higher levels. Thus, multiple levels of advocacy are needed.

MANDATE FOR A PSYCHOLOGICAL SCIENCE OF PCOS

Finally, and in addition to future interventions and advocacy, this call to action includes a mandate for psychological and other social science. A primary aim of this book is to inspire future PCOS research, particularly among psychological scientists. Notably, essential clinical research is being conducted by numerous medical researchers in the United States and internationally. However, because PCOS may potentially impact all areas of psychosocial life, more attention is especially needed on psychosocial aspects of PCOS and how these relate to health and well-being. This work might best be studied by researchers in psychology and related disciplines (e.g., sociology, public health, social work). This final section devoted to research focuses on building a psychological science of PCOS, attending to diverse PCOS experiences, and engaging the PCOS community in setting a research agenda.

We must build a psychological science of PCOS to fully understand and improve the health and well-being of individuals living with PCOS. A logical next step in building a science would be to apply existing theoretical and analytic frameworks within psychology and other related disciplines to understand PCOS and its multiple impacts more fully. One framework I put forth in this book is stigma because of its potential utility for understanding PCOS. In Chapter 2, I outlined why PCOS can be considered stigmatizing, with findings from interviews clarifying that individuals experience stigma in relation to multiple symptoms, rendering PCOS one condition with multiple stigmas. Multiple existing theoretical models of stigma supported by decades of research could be applied to understand both the experience of PCOS and its impact on the health and well-being of those living with the syndrome: weight-based stigma (Hunger et al., 2015; Sikorski et al., 2015), distinctions in stigma and multilevel contributors (Pescosolido & Martin, 2015), stigma explaining health disparities (Chaudoir et al., 2013), pathways to positive and negative outcomes of stigma (Frost, 2011), and intersecting health and identity stigmas (Stangl et al., 2019). However, I encourage psychological scientists and others to apply theories and frameworks from their own areas of psychology or related disciplines to PCOS.

This book also uncovered diverse PCOS experiences based on gender identification. Therefore, psychological science must consider potential differences and similarities in PCOS experiences in individuals with varying identities (e.g., gender, racial/ethnic). Use of an intersectionality framework in future research would encourage such consideration. Intersectionality frames experiences occurring at different intersections of social identities as stemming from societal structures and oppressions. To this end, intersectionality in psychological science on PCOS would encourage researchers to consider who is in the sample, what the similarities and differences in experience are, and how inequalities can explain them (Cole, 2009). For example, considering who is in the sample would promote recognition of individuals or groups actively left out of PCOS research. On the basis of my review of a large portion of literature for this book, PCOS research generally has been conducted with White, heterosexual, cisgender women. Also, because most PCOS research focuses on clinic-based samples, presumably what is known about PCOS is also biased toward individuals with health care access and therefore those more economically advantaged or those with U.S. citizenship. This focus may inadvertently leave out more gender diverse groups as they are less likely to have health insurance and a regular source of care than cisgender women (Gonzales & Henning-Smith, 2017). Revelation of deficient sampling and recruitment patterns could lead to more inclusive strategies: broadening language from women to individuals with PCOS, use of more inclusive images and expanded locations of advertisement. Current limited sampling in clinic settings could be replaced with broader, epidemiological approaches, which may expand representation of gender or racially diverse groups as well as those struggling economically or politically (e.g., undocumented immigrants).

In addition to diversifying samples, an intersectionality framework in PCOS psychological science would encourage deeper and contextualized understanding of PCOS experience. An intersectional lens would lead researchers to examine both similarities and differences in PCOS experiences within the population as well as compared with the population of those without PCOS and thus ground explanations of similarities and differences in inequalities (Cole, 2009). For instance, differences in experience of PCOS for individuals at varying intersections of racial/ethnic identity or gender identity might be explained by minority stress, or the identity-specific distal and proximal stressors that influence health and well-being (Meyer, 2013). This possibility fits with the health care experiences discussed in Chapter 6. Although all individuals with PCOS regardless of gender dealt with lack of PCOS knowledge, delayed diagnosis, weight bias, and dismissive behaviors from physicians, gender and racially diverse groups had the added minority stress related to racism and cultural incompetence. These intersectional experiences may be explained by structural inequalities and also undergird the reason diverse groups are less represented in clinic data.

A focus on systematic exclusion and inequalities also points to potential social determinants of health that need to be included in PCOS research. According to the U.S. Healthy People initiative aimed at setting national goals to improve population health, social determinants of health fall into five categories (economics, education, social and community context, health and health care access, and neighborhood; *Healthy People 2030*, U.S. Department of Health and Human Services, n.d.). Social determinants of health, which are grounded in inequality encountered by different identity groups, remind us that health can simultaneously be caused by and contribute to the social environment and that intermediate determinants of health (e.g., behaviors, psychosocial factors) flow from structural determinants (e.g., socioeconomic and political context; Solar & Irwin, 2010). Although I did not ask specifically about social determinants of health such as economics or health care access in the interviews I conducted, one individual, Tasha, voluntarily described access and economic challenges related to PCOS health care and particularly in the context of the COVID-19 pandemic:

> One thing that's been really difficult—finding a specialist near me. I work in rural health care, like, promotion, and so . . . I know this at an academic level, but we really are struggling to have enough providers. So, for all of my appointments, I have to drive 2 hours away to be seen. And that's difficult, especially, well, I hate driving, but that is a me problem. So, 2 hours away and then it's not covered by insurance. So, I'm currently in pretty big medical debt due to this problem, which is frustrating. And so, the pandemic kind of doubles down on that, because you aren't allowed a support person in your appointments. And so, it feels kind of isolating to drive 2 hours away, take a day off work . . . get super invasive vaginal ultrasounds and be told this is what's still wrong with you. And the appointment takes like 15 minutes, and then, it's like, "All right, bye. See you next month." And so, the pandemic has definitely, kind of, impacted that, because it's like even more isolating than normal. And of course, it was impossible to get seen for a while during the pandemic because everything was telehealth and well—telehealth can only do so much when the problem's in your gut. (*Tasha, late 20s, nonbinary*)

The bottom line is that an intersectionality framework would encourage inclusion of individuals from diverse groups living with PCOS, a nuanced understanding of PCOS experience and outcomes, as well as explanation of those within individual, social, and structural contexts. Moreover, it would incorporate additional social determinants of PCOS-related health, all of which suggest that future psychological science on PCOS should consider models of health equity (e.g., health equity promotion in LGBT people, Fredriksen-Goldsen et al., 2014; health stigmas, Stangl et al., 2019).

A final note for any future psychological science of PCOS is the need to center the lived experiences of individuals with PCOS. Excerpts from the qualitative narratives revealed many experiences never before published in scientific literature—mostly because scientists never asked about them. However, fully centering lived experience would likely mean moving away from individuals with PCOS as solely participants in research and toward individuals with PCOS as equally involved in research development, implementation, and dissemination. Community-based participatory research is one framework that can guide both researchers and communities to be equitable partners in all aspects of the research process (DiClemente et al., 2015). Integrating first-hand knowledge of PCOS held by the community with expertise in research and theory held by academics could result in research most relevant for the PCOS community and deepen understanding of PCOS (DiClemente et al., 2015).

IN SUM: A CALL TO PCOS ACTION ACROSS ECOLOGICAL SYSTEMS

Thus far, this chapter has outlined a call to action in the areas of interventions, advocacy, and psychological science to understand and improve the psychosocial impacts of PCOS. I end this chapter, and book, by emphasizing that actions toward improving the lives of individuals living with PCOS must be taken in multiple areas simultaneously. Figure 7.1 illustrates this approach, which applies an ecological model to the multiple levels at which change is needed in PCOS. Ecological models are based on the work of Urie Bronfenbrenner (1977), who argued that individuals are influenced by environments or systems nested within each other and that the impact of any one of these depends on the others. Consequently, change is needed at all these levels. Although he specifically described five systems known as micro-, meso-, exo-, macro-, and chrono-systems, I have taken a broader approach in describing related levels at which PCOS must be addressed to effect change. For example, individual-level change might entail personal growth work in individuals with PCOS to improve self-acceptance and psychological outcomes via mental health care and interventions. However, this individual work

FIGURE 7.1. Ecological Framework for Polycystic Ovary Syndrome Call to Action

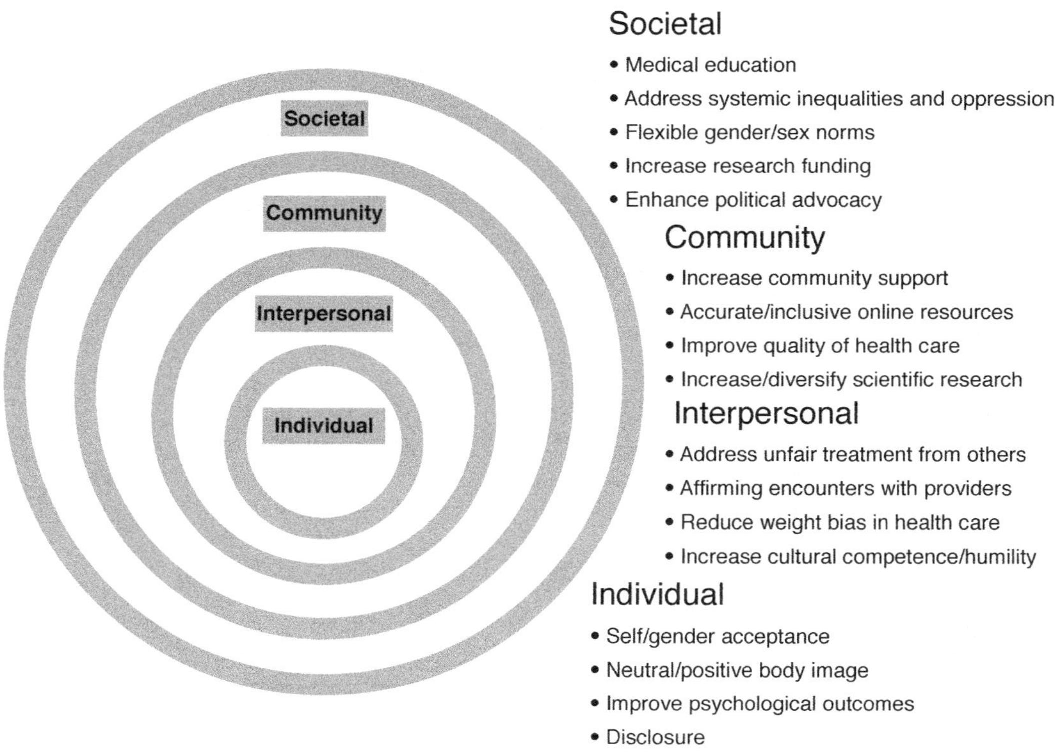

Societal

- Medical education
- Address systemic inequalities and oppression
- Flexible gender/sex norms
- Increase research funding
- Enhance political advocacy

Community

- Increase community support
- Accurate/inclusive online resources
- Improve quality of health care
- Increase/diversify scientific research

Interpersonal

- Address unfair treatment from others
- Affirming encounters with providers
- Reduce weight bias in health care
- Increase cultural competence/humility

Individual

- Self/gender acceptance
- Neutral/positive body image
- Improve psychological outcomes
- Disclosure

Societal

Community

Interpersonal

Individual

cannot be done in isolation if we want to affect the most change. Change at the interpersonal level is needed in the form of reduced discrimination or unfair treatment from others and improved and affirming provider relations (which would mean improving cultural competence and reducing weight bias among providers). Change at a community level might involve increasing available community support for PCOS, availability of accurate health resources, improved quality of care, increasing the amount of PCOS-related research, and diversifying the research being conducted.

Finally, at the social level, change would mean transforming medical education at a systems level, addressing disparities that exist, acknowledging and changing norms related to gender/sex and weight bias, increasing funding for research on PCOS, and enhancing political advocacy for these aforementioned societal changes. Visioning change via ecologically based models sheds light not only on the multiple levels that need to be addressed but also on their interconnectedness. For instance, advocacy at community or societal levels through awareness campaigns could actually reduce stigma by raising awareness in friends and family about reasons why their loved one might have facial hair or be overweight. Presumably an even broader approach such as changing societal norms to increase flexibility of expectations for gender and bodies (size, hair) could make an even larger impact to reduce stigma related to PCOS symptoms.

CONCLUSION

To summarize, the findings reported in this book should be translated into action in three main areas: interventions, advocacy, and psychological science. This change also should occur at multiple levels simultaneously to improve the psychosocial lives of individuals living with PCOS. Additionally, as this chapter concludes the book, let us return to its ultimate purpose—to address the silence surrounding PCOS and replace that silence with psychological science. As demonstrated in the first six chapters, there likely is not an aspect of psychosocial life that PCOS does not touch. The PCOS-related psychosocial experiences evidenced in the qualitative interviews are ones typically addressed in the discipline of psychology. As a social-health psychologist, an intersectional feminist, and a stigma and minority stress researcher who also has PCOS, I challenge my discipline to build a psychological science of PCOS. Further recalling the spirit of this book stated in Chapter 1, this PCOS manifesto *demands* a psychological science of PCOS that seeks to understand and ultimately reduce the full psychosocial burden of a condition that currently has no known cause or cure.

Appendix A

METHODOLOGY

SAMPLE AND RECRUITMENT

The excerpts woven throughout this book were drawn from 50 transcripts of recorded qualitative interviews I conducted between February 2020 and April 2021 by phone with individuals self-reporting a PCOS diagnosis as part of a research study titled "PCOS Stories Study." The research study was approved by the East Tennessee State University Institutional Review Board. Each interviewee received a $20 online gift card to compensate them for their time, which were funded by an internal Research Development Committee grant.

I intentionally recruited individuals from diverse groups that represented multiple racial/ethnic, gender, and sexual identities from across the United States. I recruited potential participants through advertisements on online Facebook groups focused on polycystic ovary syndrome (PCOS) and queer people with PCOS. I also advertised on Facebook and Instagram using the "boost" function, which involved paying money for the social media sites to advertise the study in people's news feeds to obtain a broader reach than what I may have gotten by the targeted advertising alone. Finally, I intentionally used images of individuals from diverse groups to recruit people of color (POC) with PCOS.

The 50 individuals living with PCOS varied in demographic characteristics as shown in Table A.1. The average age of individuals living with PCOS in the study was 29 years, and ages ranged from 19 to 46. Just over half the sample identified as gender diverse (nonbinary, genderqueer, trans; 52%), racial/ethnically diverse (54%), and either living with a partner or married (54%). Three quarters of the sample identified their sexual orientation as sexually diverse (i.e., an identity other than straight). In terms of socioeconomic

TABLE A.1. Demographic Summary of Individuals Living With Polycystic Ovary Syndrome Who Completed Interviews

Demographic characteristic	n (%)	M (SD)	Median	Min-Max
Age at interview		28.96 (6.49)	27.5	19–46
Race/ethnicity				
White non-Hispanic	23 (46%)			
Underrepresented racial/ ethnic identities[a]	27 (54%)			
Black	12 (24%)			
Hispanic	7 (14%)			
Asian	4 (8%)			
Jewish	3 (6%)			
Middle Eastern	1 (2%)			
Native American	1 (2%)			
Self-identified gender[a]				
Cisgender woman	24 (48%)			
Gender diverse	26 (52%)			
Nonbinary	20 (40%)			
Genderqueer/genderfluid	4 (8%)			
Transman/transmasculine	2 (4%)			
Self-identified sexual orientation				
Bisexual	15 (30%)			
Straight	13 (26%)			
Queer	9 (18%)			
Pansexual	6 (12%)			
Lesbian	5 (10%)			
Gay	1 (2%)			
"Indeterminately queer"	1 (2%)			
Highest education				
Bachelor's degree	18 (36%)			
Master's degree	13 (26%)			
Some college	9 (18%)			
Associate degree	4 (8%)			
High school diploma	3 (6%)			
Professional degree (JD)	1 (2%)			
Doctorate	1 (2%)			
Technical trade school	1 (2%)			
Annual income		74,489.73 (60,785.92)	65,000	14,999–400,000
Marital status				
Single	22 (44%)			
Married	16 (32%)			
Living with partner	11 (22%)			
Divorced	1 (2%)			

[a]Individuals self-reported as many identities as that applied.

indicators, the sample was more educated, with 94% of the sample having schooling beyond a high school diploma. The median income was $65,000, with incomes ranging from under $15,000 to $400,000.

ONE-ON-ONE PHONE INTERVIEWS

Individuals interested in participating clicked on a link in the advertisement that brought them to an online screener, which asked for their demographic questions and contact information. I then made contact with individuals to invite them to complete a phone interview. I used a free service (https://www.freeconferencecall.com) to complete and record the phone interviews. At the scheduled interview time, the interviewee and I both called in to the conference system. I read the informed consent document to the participant and answered any questions. Once consent was provided, I began the recording and asked a series of demographic questions followed by open-ended questions about experiences of PCOS. I asked interview questions that covered specific categories of psychosocial life to understand if and how PCOS affects their lives: how they feel about themselves and their bodies, social interactions, sexuality, gender perceptions, mental health, and health care (see Table A.2 for interview questions). I drew broadly from social psychological and health frameworks to devise interview questions that would elicit information on psychosocial impacts of PCOS. I began with questions about what interviewees believed is known by people in general about PCOS and generally followed the order of questions, although question probes were used flexibly during interviews. Afterward, I created interview notes that included notable or salient aspects of the interviewee's experiences, acknowledging my interpretation of those aspects. I used an online service (Trint) to transcribe, verbatim, the recorded interviews. Two graduate assistants edited transcripts for accuracy by comparing each transcript to the audio. I uploaded edited transcripts to NVivo 11, which I used to code transcripts during analysis.

DATA ANALYSIS

Approach

I used a reflexive thematic analysis approach to analyze the qualitative interview data (Braun & Clarke, 2006, 2022). The reflexive thematic approach values researcher subjectivity as a primary tool in qualitative analysis and

TABLE A.2. Qualitative Interview Questions

Question category	Questions

Cultural understanding of PCOS	• What do you think most people know about PCOS?
	• What don't people know about PCOS?
	  - Why do you think they don't know?
	• Do people in your life know about PCOS?
	  - Do they know about *your* PCOS?
	• How common do you think PCOS is?
	• Do you ever hear people talking about PCOS?
	  - If yes, what are they saying about it?

Personal experience	• Each person who has PCOS seems to experience it a bit differently. I would like for you to take each one of your symptoms and tell me how it affects your life. • What is the hardest thing about having PCOS? • Is there anything about your family history or your ethnicity or cultural background that you feel impacts your experience of PCOS? • What do you do to cope with your PCOS or symptoms?

Fertility	• Have you ever tried to get pregnant?
	  - If yes, did you experience any challenges due to PCOS? Can you tell me about them?
	  - If no, do you ever worry about your ability to get pregnant in the future?
	  - If yes, can you tell me about your worry?

Social impact	• How does PCOS (or symptoms of PCOS) affect your relationships?
	  - Negative or positive ways your relationships are impacted.
	  - How does PCOS impact the way you interact with other people?
	  - Does PCOS ever bring you closer to other people?
	  - Does PCOS ever drive you away from people? Or come between you and others?
	• Earlier I asked if others know about your PCOS.
	  - Can you share with me what it has been like for you to disclose your PCOS to others?
	  - If you don't disclose your PCOS to others, can you explain why you choose not to tell?
	• Do you know any other people in your life who have PCOS?
	  - Is that helpful or unhelpful?
	• Have you ever been treated differently (negatively, positively) by others because you have PCOS (or PCOS-related symptoms)?

TABLE A.2. Qualitative Interview Questions (*Continued*)

Question category	Questions

Mental health impact	• How does PCOS affect your mental health?
	  - Your happiness? Your distress level? Anxiety?
	• Have you ever sought out treatment or therapy for your mental health?
	  - Was it for reasons related to your PCOS or symptoms?
	  - What was your experience like going to therapy? Did you talk about your PCOS with your therapist? How satisfied were you with the treatment you received?

Personal impact	• How does PCOS affect the way you feel about yourself? • How does PCOS impact how you feel about your body (body image)? • Does PCOS ever make you feel "different" than other people? Or different from the way the world thinks you should be? • How does PCOS impact your dating or intimate relationships? • How does PCOS impact your sexuality? - Your satisfaction with sex?
Gender perceptions	• Does having PCOS ever make you feel more masculine or more feminine than what you want? • Do you ever feel like PCOS impacts the way you feel or think about your own gender identity? • How do you think PCOS is related to your gender? • Do you know of any people who are queer or LGBTQ who have PCOS? • How do you think PCOS might be experienced differently among people who are queer or LGBTQ?
PCOS health care	• Have you ever received treatments for your PCOS? If yes, can you explain what those treatments were or are? • Have you had any medical tests done related to your PCOS? • What were these experiences like? - How satisfied with PCOS-related health care experience are you? • How knowledgeable are your medical professionals about PCOS? • What could be better about your health care experience?
Other	• We covered a lot of topics today. What haven't we yet talked about today that you think is important for us to know about your PCOS experience? • I also recognize that we all have been experiencing a pandemic due to COVID-19. Is there anything about your PCOS that has been more challenging for you during this pandemic time? • Final question: What do you think the world needs to know about PCOS?

Note. PCOS = polycystic ovary syndrome; LGBTQ = lesbian, gay, bisexual, transgender, queer/questioning.

bases quality of analytic process and themes on reflexivity, depth of inter-pretation, and both immersion and distancing of the researcher with the data (Braun & Clarke, 2022). Because existing research and theory on PCOS are limited, I aimed to identify patterns in the psychosocial experiences reported by individuals living with PCOS. I used an overall inductive analysis process by staying as close as possible to the interview data in the development of codes and, subsequently, themes. Once code development and initial coding were complete, I immersed myself in the PCOS literature to situate themes within the literature. My prior knowledge of social psychological theories and research also informed themes to provide deeper meaning to the patterns of codes (Vaismoradi et al., 2016). Thus, whereas most of my approach involved identifying semantic or manifest meaning in the data, some latent meaning was explored during identification of themes from codes.

Process

Once edited transcripts were uploaded into NVivo 11 (QSR International, 2015), I read each transcript and developed preliminary codes, which I then used to code remaining transcripts. During this iterative process, some codes were merged, and others were split into different codes. I used the list of codes to code transcripts systematically in NVivo to enhance consistency of coding and cohesion in process and themes and, therefore, rigor of quali-tative analysis (Roberts et al., 2019). Although reflexive thematic analysis does not involve reaching consensus between multiple coders, collaborative aspects of coding can be used to enhance reflexivity and understanding (Braun & Clarke, 2022). As such, I employed collaborative coding strategies during code development and the coding process. Specifically, I enlisted the assistance of two doctoral-level graduate research assistants unaware of PCOS research. One assistant read a subset of transcripts and created a unique list of codes to which I compared mine before finalizing the codes. The other assis-tant coded a random 20% ($n = 10$) of transcripts, and together we discussed coded transcripts and implementation of the coding scheme before finalizing themes. I sought these discussions about the data with individuals not expert in PCOS to provide additional depth to my own coding and analysis process.

During analysis, I alternated between reading PCOS and other literature and developing themes both to immerse myself in and to distance myself from the data. This cyclic process allowing distance from the data promotes congruence between the study purpose (i.e., in this case, a descriptive study of psychosocial experiences of PCOS) and data analysis. This cycle allows the researcher, regardless of whether coding occurs by one researcher or involves group discussion, to reenter the data with a new perspective (Vaismoradi et al., 2016). I subsequently identified themes by organizing codes based on similarity of meaning across all interview question categories. These themes that summarize psychosocial experiences became the chapters of this book, as depicted in Table A.3. Discussion of findings in the book is grounded in lived experience, as illustrated by my heavy use of excerpts from the interview transcripts. Because the participants are not a representative sample of the population of individuals with PCOS, it is not necessary to consider frequency

TABLE A.3. Psychosocial Experiences of PCOS by Theme

Theme	Psychosocial experience
Silence surrounding PCOS	PCOS as invisible condition
	Invisibility of gender-diverse experience
	Invisibility of culturally diverse experiences
	Cultural disregard for female issues
	Understanding limited to infertility
PCOS stigma	Internalized stigma attached to symptoms
	Enacted stigma
Gendered embodiment of PCOS	Body-related dysphoria
	Threatened womanhood
	Negative body image
	Feeling less attractive/desirable
	PCOS concordant with gender
	PCOS as asset for gender identity
	PCOS as intersex condition
Close relationship processes	Pressure to conform/social control
	Support/positive impact
	Lack of PCOS support
	Concealment/disclosure
	Partner/dating impact
	Avoidance of sex due to negative body image
	Increased libido
Psychological symptoms and growth	Negative impact of PCOS
	Resilience/psychological growth
	Mental health care encounters
Inadequate health care resources	Lack of knowledge about PCOS
	Delayed diagnosis
	Dismissive health care experiences
	Weight bias in medical setting
	Lack of cultural competence in health care
	What positive health care encounters look like

Note. PCOS = polycystic ovary syndrome.

of reported codes and themes; frequency does not equate to importance (Braun & Clarke, 2006). I considered with great care the ethical issue of confidentiality when choosing these excerpts and associated demographics to report (Braun & Clarke, 2022). Additionally, I chose pseudonyms for all participants and omitted or disguised idiosyncratic details as much possible so as not to identify participants indirectly. For additional protection to avoid identification, age range and gender were specified but not race/ethnicity for all excerpts. Instead, participant demographics were presented in aggregate in Table A.1.

More on Reflexivity
In addition to reflexivity as acknowledgment of how methodological decisions and disciplinary knowledge plays a role in analysis, personal reflexivity explores how researcher values shape understanding of the knowledge produced (Wilkinson, 1988). Throughout the research process, including the development of the interview questions, the recruitment of participants, the interview process, and analysis of transcripts, I intentionally and continually maintained awareness of my positionality in relation to the research. This reflects the value of transparency in qualitative research (Levitt et al., 2018). As a woman with PCOS for 30 years, I would be considered an insider (someone with PCOS studying PCOS) versus outsider (someone without PCOS studying PCOS) researcher, both of which can come with benefits and pitfalls (Hayfield & Huxley, 2015). Insider status obviously gave me insight into the condition and the types of symptoms and experiences to ask about. Yet because of the diverse symptoms of PCOS, I may be considered an outsider based on symptoms that I do not encounter and therefore was not attuned to ask about. Two specific examples come to mind. First, individuals I initially interviewed mentioned experiencing pain as a result of PCOS when I asked if there were any symptoms that they encounter that I did not list. Most likely because my own experience of PCOS does not involve pain, I did not include it in the list of PCOS symptoms. Second, because I am a White woman, I was not initially considering how culture or ethnic identity could interact with PCOS experience. Thus, I added questions that directly asked about PCOS-related pain and that captured ways that cultural or ethnic background impact PCOS experience. Still, my own majority racial/ethnic identity may have limited what individuals shared about cultural impact.

My identity as a lesbian and queer White woman with PCOS influenced my recruitment of particular demographics of participants that I needed to address. My personal identities influenced my participation in online Facebook groups focused on queer individuals with PCOS which played a role in participant recruitment. Additionally, my own race/ethnicity could have contributed to my recruitment of mostly White participants initially. Because it was important to me to represent the range of individuals that experience PCOS, I intentionally recruited people of color with PCOS with advertisements featuring individuals of varying race/ethnicity. Fortunately, this intentional advertising resulted in recruiting people of color, although of course these qualitative data are not intended to represent or generalize to all individuals with PCOS.

Additionally, although I believe I have included a diverse set of voices within this book, there remains a lack of inclusion of individuals aged 45 and older with PCOS and individuals under age 18. Older individuals were most likely not recruited because of issues related to the timing of diagnosis but also possibly due to generational differences in the use of social media or online support groups. This limitation may be particularly noteworthy given the major health implications of PCOS over time—its association with chronic and serious morbidities such as heart disease and diabetes. I purposefully did not recruit minors for this project, focusing my interviews on adults only so that a parental permission process was not involved. Adolescents with PCOS are an important age group to study given that their psychosocial experiences would be currently experienced rather than retrospectively reported in research studies.

In addition to a limited age range, all the individuals I interviewed had at least a high school diploma, and many of them had college or even graduate degrees. The number of individuals with PCOS of any age who have less than a high school education is unknown, and therefore their experiences are unknown. And, although I included questions about gender and sexual identity, the relationship orientation of all individuals is unknown. A couple of interviewees mentioned that they were polyamorous; whereas they may have been legally married to one partner, they had other partners as well. I did not explicitly ask all interviewees to report relationship orientation, however. Perhaps more important, as a result, representation of the social and sexual impact of PCOS in the book likely does not fully capture the full range of experiences. Because this is a common deficit in the psychological literature, I believe much more attention needs to be paid to the relationship orientation of our research participants.

MORE ON DATA COLLECTION DURING THE COVID-19 PANDEMIC

Interviews for the PCOS Stories Study were conducted from February 2020 to May 2021. Shortly after initiating data collection, the COVID-19 pandemic began. As such, the bulk of the interviews with individuals living with PCOS took place during the pandemic. During a period of 4 months, from March until July 2020, I halted data collection to avoid causing undue stress to participants during the initial time of the pandemic when life seemed especially uncertain. When I resumed data collection, I modified the interview protocol to include a final question asking about how COVID-19 may have influenced their experience of PCOS. Responses to the question about the impact of the pandemic on PCOS ranged from no impact to descriptions of health care access challenges to improved satisfaction with health care to mental health challenges from anxiety and social isolation to positive implications of masks hiding facial hair.

SUGGESTED READING LIST

For more in-depth consideration of polycystic ovary syndrome (PCOS) and the various psychosocial aspects of life discussed in this book, I recommend these readings. They are a mixture of medical, social science, and popular press sources that contributed to the growth of my own knowledge in these areas and in relation to PCOS.

Azziz, R., Nestler, J. E., & Dewailly, D. (2006). *Androgen excess disorders in women: Polycystic ovary syndrome and other disorders* (2nd ed.). Humana Press.
This edited text provides technical medical understanding of PCOS and other disorders due to androgen excess.

Barry, J. A. (2019). *Psychological aspects of polycystic ovary syndrome*. Palgrave MacMillan.
This book addresses psychological aspects of PCOS through a lens of the impact of androgens, insulin, and stress.

Block, J. (2019). *Everything below the waist: Why health care needs a feminist revolution*. St. Martin's Press.
This book demands a revolution in health care for women, weaving together historical accounts and health care experiences.

Bobel, C., & Kwan, S. (2011). *Embodied resistance: Changing the norms, breaking the rules*. Vanderbilt University Press.
An anthology about negotiating embodiment and identity focused on sexuality, gender, and race.

Brown, B. (2007). *I thought it was just me (but it isn't): Making the journey from "what will people think?" to "I am enough."* Avery, Penguin Random House.
A popular press book focused on the universal experience of shame.

Chrisler, J. C., & Johnston-Robledo, I. (2019). *Woman's embodied self: Feminist perspectives on identity and image*. American Psychological Association.
This text offers a deep understanding of the connections between women's bodies and their self-identities through a feminist and cultural lens. This book

is complementary to the current book for its in-depth dive into body image and societal expectations.

Collins, P. H. (2019). *Intersectionality as critical social theory*. Duke University Press. A critical text that encourages movement of intersectionality into the realm of social theory.

Collins, P. H., & Bilge, S. (2016). *Intersectionality*. Polity. A foundational text on intersectionality.

Fahs, B. (2020). *Burn it down! Feminist manifestos for the revolution*. Verso Books. A collection of feminist manifestos to inspire change.

Fausto-Sterling, A. (2020). *Sexing the body: Gender politics and the construction of sexuality*. Hachette Book Group. A revolutionary text exploring the body in societal and political context, with a focus on gender identity and intersex people.

Goffman, E. (1963). *Stigma: Notes on the management of spoiled identity*. Simon & Schuster. A foundation of stigma theory essential for understanding stigma. Warning: uses original outdated language that is offensive and reminds us of the historical context in which stigma theory was developed and therefore how far we have come.

Malatino, H. (2019). *Queer embodiment: Monstrosity, medical violence, and intersex experience*. University of Nebraska Press. This groundbreaking book takes a critical eye to the treatment of intersexuality by integrating archival research, personal account, and theory.

Neff, K. (2021). *Fierce self-compassion: How women can harness kindness to speak up, claim their power, and thrive*. HarperCollins. An application of her groundbreaking self-compassion research to women's experience in modern culture.

Park, C. L., Lechner, S. C., Antoni, M. H., & Stanton, A. L. (2009). *Medical illness and positive life change: Can crisis lead to personal transformation?* American Psychological Association. This edited volume provides perspectives on ways that individuals can emerge from health-related crises in ways that reflect growth and meaning in life.

Perez, C. C. (2019). *Invisible women: Data bias in a world designed for men*. Abrams Press. A book that explores the gender inequalities that stem from gender bias in data.

Petersen, J. K. (2021). *A comprehensive guide to intersex*. Jessica Kingsley Publishers. A resource providing information on more than 40 variations, as well as history and medical interventions.

Rajunov, M., & Duane, S. (2019). *Nonbinary memoirs of gender and identity*. Columbia University Press. An anthology of essays capturing nonbinary gender experiences in a gender binary world.

Serano, J. (2016). *Whipping girl: A transsexual woman on sexism and the scapegoating of femininity*. Seal Press.

A provocative view of transgender identities that integrates theory, personal essay, and manifesto.

Stryker, S. (2008). *Transgender history: The roots of today's revolution*. Seal Press.

A thorough text on trans history and activism.

Taylor, S. R. (2018). *The body is not an apology: The power of radical self-love*. Berrett-Koehler Publishers.

A radical book to encourage self-love and breaking free from body shame.

Thatcher, S. S. (2000). *Polycystic ovary syndrome: The hidden epidemic*. Perspectives Press.

Although this text is older, it provides a comprehensive understanding of PCOS and its impacts through the lens of a health care provider and endocrinologist who specialized in PCOS. Chapter 6 offers suggestions on how to find adequate health care providers in PCOS. Chapter 10 is written by Dr. Melissa Himelein, who covers ways to resist body shaming in PCOS.

Viloria, H. (2017). *Born both: An intersex life*. Hachette Books.

An autobiographical account of intersexuality by an intersex activist.

Viloria, H., & Nieto, M. (2020). *The spectrum of sex: The science of male, female, and intersex*. Jessica Kingsley Publishers.

A helpful guide to understanding sex and gender identity, the gender binary, and intersex variation.

References

Abdollahi, L., Mirghafourvand, M., Kheyradin, J. B., & Mohammadi, M. (2019). Effectiveness of cognitive-behavioral therapy (CBT) in improving the quality of life and psychological fatigue in women with polycystic ovarian syndrome: A randomized controlled clinical trial. *Journal of Psychosomatic Obstetrics & Gynecology*, *40*(4), 283–293. https://doi.org/10.1080/0167482X.2018.1502265

Alberga, A. S., Edache, I. Y., Forhan, M., & Russell-Mayhew, S. (2019). Weight bias and health care utilization: A scoping review. *Primary Health Care Research and Development*, *20*(e116), e116. https://doi.org/10.1017/S1463423619000227

Alberga, A. S., Pickering, B. J., Alix Hayden, K., Ball, G. D. C., Edwards, A., Jelinski, S., Nutter, S., Oddie, S., Sharma, A. M., & Russell-Mayhew, S. (2016). Weight bias reduction in health professionals: A systematic review. *Clinical Obesity*, *6*(3), 175–188. https://doi.org/10.1111/cob.12147

Alur-Gupta, S., Chemerinski, A., Liu, C., Lipson, J., Allison, K., Sammel, M. D., & Dokras, A. (2019). Body-image distress is increased in women with polycystic ovary syndrome and mediates depression and anxiety. *Fertility and Sterility*, *112*(5), 930–938.e1. https://doi.org/10.1016/j.fertnstert.2019.06.018

Alur-Gupta, S., Lee, I., Chemerinski, A., Liu, C., Lipson, J., Allison, K., Gallop, R., & Dokras, A. (2021). Racial differences in anxiety, depression, and quality of life in women with polycystic ovary syndrome. *Fertility & Sterility Report*, *2*, 2666–3341. https://doi.org/10.1016/j.xfre.2021.03.003

American Psychiatric Association. (2013). *Diagnostic and statistical manual of mental disorders* (5th ed.). https://doi.org/10.1176/appi.books.9780890425596

American Psychological Association. (2015). *Key terms and concepts in understanding gender diversity and sexual orientation among students*. https://www.apa.org/pi/lgbt/programs/safe-supportive/lgbt/key-terms.pdf

Amiri, N. F., Ramezani Tehrani, F., Simbar, M., Mohammadpour Thamtan, R. A., & Shiva, N. (2014). Female gender scheme is disturbed by polycystic ovary syndrome: A qualitative study from Iran. *Iranian Red Crescent Medical Journal*, *16*(2), e12423. https://doi.org/10.5812/ircmj.12423

Amiri, N. F., Ramezani Tehrani, F., Simbar, M., Montazeri, A., & Mohammadpour, R. A. (2016). Health-related quality of life questionnaire for polycystic ovary syndrome (PCOSQ-50): Development and psychometric properties. *Quality of Life Research, 25*(7), 1791–1801. https://doi.org/10.1007/s11136-016-1232-7

Ananthakumar, T., Jones, N. R., Hinton, L., & Aveyard, P. (2020). Clinical encounters about obesity: Systematic review of patients' perspectives. *Clinical Obesity, 10*(1), e12347. https://doi.org/10.1111/cob.12347

Arroyo, A., Burke, T. J., & Young, V. J. (2020). The role of close others in promoting weight management and body image outcomes: An application of confirmation, self-determination, social control, and social support. *Journal of Social and Personal Relationships, 37*(3), 1030–1050. https://doi.org/10.1177/0265407519886066

Ashwell, M., Gunn, P., & Gibson, S. (2012). Waist-to-height ratio is a better screening tool than waist circumference and BMI for adult cardiometabolic risk factors: Systematic review and meta-analysis. *Obesity Reviews, 13*(3), 275–286. https://doi.org/10.1111/j.1467-789X.2011.00952.x

Association for Size Diversity and Health. (n.d.). *HAES principles*. https://asdah.org/health-at-every-size-haes-approach/

Austin, A., & Goodman, R. (2018). Perceptions of transition-related health and mental health services among transgender adults. *Journal of Gay & Lesbian Social Services, 30*(1), 17–32. https://doi.org/10.1080/10538720.2017.1408515

Azziz, R. (2016). Introduction: Determinants of polycystic ovary syndrome. *Fertility and Sterility, 106*(1), 4–5. https://doi.org/10.1016/j.fertnstert.2016.05.009

Azziz, R. (2018). Polycystic ovary syndrome. *Obstetrics and Gynecology, 132*(2), 321–336. https://doi.org/10.1097/AOG.0000000000002698

Azziz, R., Carmina, E., Dewailly, D., Diamanti-Kandarakis, E., Escobar-Morreale, H. F., Futterweit, W., Janssen, O. E., Legro, R. S., Norman, R. J., Taylor, A. E., Witchel, S. F., & the Task Force on the Phenotype of the Polycystic Ovary Syndrome of the Androgen Excess and PCOS Society. (2009). The Androgen Excess and PCOS Society criteria for the polycystic ovary syndrome: The complete task force report. *Fertility and Sterility, 91*(2), 456–488. https://doi.org/10.1016/j.fertnstert.2008.06.035

Azziz, R., Dumesic, D. A., & Goodarzi, M. O. (2011). Polycystic ovary syndrome: An ancient disorder? *Fertility and Sterility, 95*(5), 1544–1548. https://doi.org/10.1016/j.fertnstert.2010.09.032

Azziz, R., Woods, K. S., Reyna, R., Key, T. J., Knochenhauer, E. S., & Yildiz, B. O. (2004). The prevalence and features of the polycystic ovary syndrome in an unselected population. *The Journal of Clinical Endocrinology and Metabolism, 89*(6), 2745–2749. https://doi.org/10.1210/jc.2003-032046

Baba, T., Endo, T., Ikeda, K., Shimizu, A., Honnma, H., Ikeda, H., Masumori, N., Ohmura, T., Kiya, T., Fujimoto, T., Koizumi, M., & Saito, T. (2011). Distinctive features of female-to-male transsexualism and prevalence of gender identity disorder in Japan. *Journal of Sexual Medicine, 8*(6), 1686–1693. https://doi.org/10.1111/j.1743-6109.2011.02252.x

Bacon, L., Stern, J. S., Van Loan, M. D., & Keim, N. L. (2005). Size acceptance and intuitive eating improve health for obese, female chronic dieters. *Journal of the American Dietetic Association, 105*(6), 929–936. https://doi.org/10.1016/j.jada.2005.03.011

Balani, J., Hyer, S., Wagner, M., & Shehata, H. (2013). Obesity, polycystic ovaries and impaired reproductive outcome. In T. A. Mahmood & S. Arulkumaran (Eds.), *Obesity: A ticking time bomb for reproductive health* (pp. 289–298). Elsevier. https://doi.org/10.1016/B978-0-12-416045-3.00022-4

Barnard, L., Ferriday, D., Guenther, N., Strauss, B., Balen, A. H., & Dye, L. (2007). Quality of life and psychological well being in polycystic ovary syndrome. *Human Reproduction, 22*(8), 2279–2286. https://doi.org/10.1093/humrep/dem108

Barrera, M., Jr. (1986). Distinctions between social support concepts, measures, and models. *American Journal of Community Psychology, 14*(4), 413–445. https://doi.org/10.1007/BF00922627

Barry, J. A. (2019). *Psychological aspects of polycystic ovary syndrome.* Palgrave MacMillan. https://doi.org/10.1007/978-3-030-30290-0

Barth, J. H., Catalan, J., Cherry, C. A., & Day, A. (1993). Psychological morbidity in women referred for treatment of hirsutism. *Journal of Psychosomatic Research, 37*(6), 615–619. https://doi.org/10.1016/0022-3999(93)90056-L

Bartholomew, M. W., Harris, A. N., & Maglalang, D. D. (2018). A call to healing: Black Lives Matter movement as a framework for addressing the health and wellness of Black women. *Community Psychology in Global Perspective, 4,* 85–100. https://doi.org/10.1285/i24212113v4i2p85

Bazarganipour, F., Ziaei, S., Montazeri, A., Foroozanfard, F., Kazemnejad, A., & Faghihzadeh, S. (2013). Predictive factors of health-related quality of life in patients with polycystic ovary syndrome: A structural equation modeling approach. *Fertility and Sterility, 100*(5), 1389–1396. https://doi.org/10.1016/j.fertnstert.2013.06.043

Bazarganipour, F., Ziaei, S., Montazeri, A., Foroozanfard, F., Kazemnejad, A., & Faghihzadeh, S. (2014). Health-related quality of life in patients with polycystic ovary syndrome (PCOS): A model-based study of predictive factors. *Journal of Sexual Medicine, 11*(4), 1023–1032. https://doi.org/10.1111/jsm.12405

Becker, G., & Nachtigall, R. D. (1994). "Born to be a mother": The cultural construction of risk in infertility treatment in the U.S. *Social Science & Medicine, 39*(4), 507–518. https://doi.org/10.1016/0277-9536(94)90093-0

Ben, J., Cormack, D., Harris, R., & Paradies, Y. (2017). Racism and health service utilisation: A systematic review and meta-analysis. *PLOS ONE, 12*(12), e0189900. https://doi.org/10.1371/journal.pone.0189900

Block, J. (2019). *Everything below the waist: Why health care needs a feminist revolution.* St. Martin's Press.

Blodorn, A., Major, B., Hunger, J., & Miller, C. (2016). Unpacking the psychological weight of weight stigma: A rejection-expectation pathway. *Journal of Experimental Social Psychology, 63*, 69–76. https://doi.org/10.1016/j.jesp.2015.12.003

Bockting, W. O. (2009). Transforming the paradigm of transgender health: A field in transition. *Sexual and Relationship Therapy, 24*(2), 103–107. https://doi.org/10.1080/14681990903037660

Bonner, A., Yadav, S., Delau, O., Markovic, D., Patterson, W., Ottey, S., & Azziz, R. (2022, June). *Direct costs of mental health disorders in PCOS: Systematic review and meta-analysis* [Poster presentation]. The 104th Annual Meeting of the Endocrine Society, Atlanta, GA, United States.

Borghi, L., Leone, D., Vegni, E., Galiano, V., Lepadatu, C., Sulpizio, P., & Garzia, E. (2018). Psychological distress, anger and quality of life in polycystic ovary syndrome: Associations with biochemical, phenotypical and socio-demographic factors. *Journal of Psychosomatic Obstetrics and Gynaecology, 39*(2), 128–137. https://doi.org/10.1080/0167482X.2017.1311319

Boudreau, D., Mukerjee, R., Wesp, L., & Letcher, L. N. (2021). Trauma-informed care. In R. Mukerjee, L. Wesp, R. Singer, & D. Menkin (Eds.), *Clinician's guide to LGBTQIA+ care: Cultural safety and social justice in primary, sexual, and reproductive healthcare* (pp. 69–81). Springer. https://doi.org/10.1891/9780826169211.0005

Bowleg, L. (2008). When Black + lesbian + women ≠ Black lesbian woman: The methodological challenges of qualitative and quantitative intersectionality research. *Sex Roles, 59*(5–6), 312–325. https://doi.org/10.1007/s11199-008-9400-z

Bozdag, G., Mumusoglu, S., Zengin, D., Karabulut, E., & Yildiz, B. O. (2016). The prevalence and phenotypic features of polycystic ovary syndrome: A systematic review and meta-analysis. *Human Reproduction, 31*(12), 2841–2855. https://doi.org/10.1093/humrep/dew218

Brakta, S., Lizneva, D., Mykhalchenko, K., Imam, A., Walker, W., Diamond, M. P., & Azziz, R. (2017). Perspectives on polycystic ovary syndrome: Is polycystic ovary syndrome research underfunded? *The Journal of Clinical Endocrinology and Metabolism, 102*(12), 4421–4427. https://doi.org/10.1210/jc.2017-01415

Braun, V., & Clarke, V. (2006). Using thematic analysis in psychology. *Qualitative Research in Psychology, 3*(2), 77–101. https://doi.org/10.1191/1478088706qp063oa

Braun, V., & Clarke, V. (2022). Conceptual and design thinking for thematic analysis. *Qualitative Psychology, 9*(1), 3–26. https://doi.org/10.1037/qup0000196

Bronfenbrenner, U. (1977). Toward an experimental ecology of human development. *American Psychologist, 32*(7), 513–531. https://doi.org/10.1037/0003-066X.32.7.513

Bronfenbrenner, U. (1979). *The ecology of human development: Experiments by nature and design.* Harvard University Press.

Brown, B. (2007). *I thought it was just me (but it isn't): Making the journey from "what will people think?" to "I am enough".* Penguin Random House.

Brunson, J. A., Overup, C. S., Nguyen, M. L., Novak, S. A., & Smith, C. V. (2014). Good intentions gone awry? Effects of weight-related social control on health and well-being. *Body Image, 11*(1), 1–10. https://doi.org/10.1016/j.bodyim.2013.08.003

Brutocao, C., Zaiem, F., Alsawas, M., Morrow, A. S., Murad, M. H., & Javed, A. (2018). Psychiatric disorders in women with polycystic ovary syndrome: A systematic review and meta-analysis. *Endocrine, 62*(2), 318–325. https://doi.org/10.1007/s12020-018-1692-3

Buchanan, N. T., Rios, D., & Case, K. A. (2020). Intersectional cultural humility: Aligning critical inquiry with critical praxis in psychology. *Women & Therapy, 43*(3–4), 235–243. https://doi.org/10.1080/02703149.2020.1729469

Butler, J. (1990). *Gender trouble.* Routledge.

Callan, V. J. (1985). Perceptions of parents, the voluntarily and involuntarily childless: A multidimensional scaling analysis. *Journal of Marriage and Family, 47*(4), 1045–1050. https://doi.org/10.2307/352349

Carmina, E. (2004). Diagnosis of polycystic ovary syndrome: From NIH criteria to ESHRE-ASRM guidelines. *Minerva Ginecologica, 56*(1), 1–6.

Carmina, E., & Lobo, R. A. (1999). Polycystic ovary syndrome (PCOS): Arguably the most common endocrinopathy is associated with significant morbidity in women. *The Journal of Clinical Endocrinology and Metabolism, 84*(6), 1897–1899. https://doi.org/10.1210/jcem.84.6.5803

Chaudhari, A. P., Mazumdar, K., & Mehta, P. D. (2018). Anxiety, depression, and quality of life in women with polycystic ovary syndrome. *Indian Journal of Psychological Medicine, 40*(3), 239–246. https://doi.org/10.4103/IJPSYM.IJPSYM_561_17

Chaudoir, S. R., Earnshaw, V. A., & Andel, S. (2013). "Discredited" versus "discreditable": Understanding how shared and unique stigma mechanisms affect psychological and physical health disparities. *Basic and Applied Social Psychology, 35*(1), 75–87. https://doi.org/10.1080/01973533.2012.746612

Chaudoir, S. R., Wang, K., & Pachankis, J. E. (2017). What reduces sexual minority stress? A review of the intervention "toolkit." *Journal of Social Issues, 73*(3), 586–617. https://doi.org/10.1111/josi.12233

Chrisler, J. C. (2011). Leaks, lumps, and lines: Stigma and women's bodies. *Psychology of Women Quarterly, 35*(2), 202–214. https://doi.org/10.1177/0361684310397698

Chrisler, J. C., Gorman, J. A., Manion, J., Murgo, M., Barney, A., Adams-Clark, A., Newton, J. R., & McGrath, M. (2016). Queer periods: Attitudes toward and experiences with menstruation in the masculine of centre and transgender community. *Culture, Health & Sexuality, 18*(11), 1238–1250. https://doi.org/10.1080/13691058.2016.1182645

Chrisler, J. C., & Johnston-Robledo, I. (2018). *Woman's embodied self: Feminist perspectives on identity and image.* American Psychological Association. https://doi.org/10.1037/0000047-000

Chrisler, J. C., & Zittel, C. B. (1998). Menarche stories: Reminiscences of college students from Lithuania, Malaysia, Sudan, and the United States. *Health Care for Women International, 19*(4), 303–312. https://doi.org/10.1080/073993398246287

Clifford, D., Ozier, A., Bundros, J., Moore, J., Kreiser, A., & Morris, M. N. (2015). Impact of non-diet approaches on attitudes, behaviors, and health outcomes: A systematic review. *Journal of Nutrition Education and Behavior, 47*(2), 143–55.e1. https://doi.org/10.1016/j.jneb.2014.12.002

Cohen, S., Underwood, L. G., & Gottlieb, B. H. (Eds.). (2000). *Social support measurement and intervention: A guide for health and social scientists.* Oxford University Press. https://doi.org/10.1093/med:psych/9780195126709.001.0001

Cole, E. R. (2009). Intersectionality and research in psychology. *American Psychologist, 64*(3), 170–180. https://doi.org/10.1037/a0014564

Collins, P. H. (2019). *Intersectionality as critical social theory.* Duke University Press.

Conte, F., Banting, L., Teede, H. J., & Stepto, N. K. (2015). Mental health and physical activity in women with polycystic ovary syndrome: A brief review. *Sports Medicine, 45*(4), 497–504. https://doi.org/10.1007/s40279-014-0291-6

Cooney, L. G., & Dokras, A. (2018). Beyond fertility: Polycystic ovary syndrome and long-term health. *Fertility and Sterility, 110*(5), 794–809. https://doi.org/10.1016/j.fertnstert.2018.08.021

Cooney, L. G., Lee, I., Sammel, M. D., & Dokras, A. (2017). High prevalence of moderate and severe depressive and anxiety symptoms in polycystic ovary syndrome: A systematic review and meta-analysis. *Human Reproduction, 32*(5), 1075–1091. https://doi.org/10.1093/humrep/dex044

Cooney, L. G., Milman, L. W., Hantsoo, L., Kornfield, S., Sammel, M. D., Allison, K. C., Epperson, C. N., & Dokras, A. (2018). Cognitive-behavioral therapy improves weight loss and quality of life in women with polycystic ovary syndrome: A pilot randomized clinical trial. *Fertility and Sterility, 110*(1), 161–171.e1. https://doi.org/10.1016/j.fertnstert.2018.03.028

Crenshaw, K. (1989). Demarginalizing the intersection of race and sex: A Black feminist critique of antidiscrimination doctrine, feminist theory and antiracist politics. *University of Chicago Legal Forum, 1989,* 139–167.

Crete, J., & Adamshick, P. (2011). Managing polycystic ovary syndrome: What our patients are telling us. *Journal of Holistic Nursing, 29*(4), 256–266. https://doi.org/10.1177/0898010111398660

Crocker, J., Major, B., & Steele, C. (1998). Social stigma. In D. T. Gilbert & S. T. Fiske (Eds.), *The handbook of social psychology* (pp. 504–553). McGraw-Hill.

Cronin, L., Guyatt, G., Griffith, L., Wong, E., Azziz, R., Futterweit, W., Cook, D., & Dunaif, A. (1998). Development of a health-related quality-of-life questionnaire (PCOSQ) for women with polycystic ovary syndrome (PCOS). *The Journal of Clinical Endocrinology and Metabolism, 83*(6), 1976–1987. https://doi.org/10.1210/jcem.83.6.4990

Damone, A. L., Joham, A. E., Loxton, D., Earnest, A., Teede, H. J., & Moran, L. J. (2019). Depression, anxiety and perceived stress in women with and without PCOS: A community-based study. *Psychological Medicine, 49*(9), 1510–1520. https://doi.org/10.1017/S0033291718002076

de Ridder, C. M., Bruning, P. F., Zonderland, M. L., Thijssen, J. H. H., Bonfrer, J. M. G., Blankenstein, M. A., Huisveld, I. A., & Erich, W. B. M. (1990). Body fat mass, body fat distribution, and plasma hormones in early puberty in females. *The Journal of Clinical Endocrinology and Metabolism, 70*(4), 888–893. https://doi.org/10.1210/jcem-70-4-888

DeUgarte, C. M., Woods, K. S., Bartolucci, A. A., & Azziz, R. (2006). Degree of facial and body terminal hair growth in unselected Black and White women: Toward a populational definition of hirsutism. *The Journal of Clinical Endocrinology and Metabolism, 91*, 1345–1350. https://doi.org/10.1210/jc.2004-2301

Diamanti-Kandarakis, E., Kouli, C. R., Bergiele, A. T., Filandra, F. A., Tsianateli, T. C., Spina, G. G., Zapanti, E. D., & Bartzis, M. I. (1999). A survey of the polycystic ovary syndrome in the Greek island of Lesbos: Hormonal and metabolic profile. *The Journal of Clinical Endocrinology and Metabolism, 84*(11), 4006–4011. https://doi.org/10.1210/jcem.84.11.6148

DiClemente, R. J., Salazar, L. F., & Crosby, R. A. (2015). Community-based participatory research in the context of health promotion. In L. F. Salazar, R. A. Crosby, & R. J. DiClemente (Eds.), *Research methods in health promotion* (pp. 313–335). John Wiley & Sons.

Dokras, A. (2012). Mood and anxiety disorders in women with PCOS. *Steroids, 77*(4), 338–341. https://doi.org/10.1016/j.steroids.2011.12.008

Dokras, A., Bochner, M., Hollinrake, E., Markham, S., Vanvoorhis, B., & Jagasia, D. H. (2005). Screening women with polycystic ovary syndrome for metabolic syndrome. *Obstetrics and Gynecology, 106*(1), 131–137. https://doi.org/10.1097/01.AOG.0000167408.30893.6b

Dokras, A., Clifton, S., Futterweit, W., & Wild, R. (2011). Increased risk for abnormal depression scores in women with polycystic ovary syndrome: A systematic review and meta-analysis. *Obstetrics and Gynecology, 117*(1), 145–152. https://doi.org/10.1097/AOG.0b013e318202b0a4

Dokras, A., Clifton, S., Futterweit, W., & Wild, R. (2012). Increased prevalence of anxiety symptoms in women with polycystic ovary syndrome: Systematic review and meta-analysis. *Fertility and Sterility, 97*(1), 225–30.e2. https://doi.org/10.1016/j.fertnstert.2011.10.022

Dokras, A., Stener-Victorin, E., Yildiz, B. O., Li, R., Ottey, S., Shah, D., Epperson, N., & Teede, H. (2018). Androgen Excess-Polycystic Ovary Syndrome Society: Position statement on depression, anxiety, quality of life, and eating disorders in polycystic ovary syndrome. *Fertility and Sterility, 109*(5), 888–899. https://doi.org/10.1016/j.fertnstert.2018.01.038

Dokras, A., & Witchel, S. F. (2014). Are young adult women with polycystic ovary syndrome slipping through the healthcare cracks? *The Journal of Clinical*

Endocrinology and Metabolism, 99(5), 1583–1585. https://doi.org/10.1210/jc.2013-4190

Duggan, A. P. (2019). *Health and illness in close relationships. Advances in personal relationships*. Cambridge University Press. https://doi.org/10.1017/9781108325578

Dupras, D. M., Wieland, M. L., Halvorsen, A. J., Maldonado, M., Willett, L. L., & Harris, L. (2020). Assessment of training in health disparities in US Internal Medicine Residency Programs. *JAMA Network Open, 3*(8), e2012757. https://doi.org/10.1001/jamanetworkopen.2020.12757

Ee, C., Smith, C., Moran, L., MacMillan, F., Costello, M., Baylock, B., & Teede, H. (2020). "The whole package deal": Experiences of overweight/obese women living with polycystic ovary syndrome. *BMC Women's Health, 20*(1), 221. https://doi.org/10.1186/s12905-020-01090-7

Eftekhar, T., Sohrabvand, F., Zabandan, N., Shariat, M., Haghollahi, F., & Ghahghaei-Nezamabadi, A. (2014). Sexual dysfunction in patients with polycystic ovary syndrome and its affected domains. *Iranian Journal of Reproductive Medicine, 12*(8), 539–546.

Eger, E. (2020). *The gift: 12 lessons to save your life*. Scribner.

Elsenbruch, S., Hahn, S., Kowalsky, D., Offner, A. H., Schedlowski, M., Mann, K., & Janssen, O. E. (2003). Quality of life, psychosocial well-being, and sexual satisfaction in women with polycystic ovary syndrome. *The Journal of Clinical Endocrinology and Metabolism, 88*(12), 5801–5807. https://doi.org/10.1210/jc.2003-030562

Elson, J. (2004). *Am I still a woman? Hysterectomy and gender identity*. Temple University Press.

Evers, A. W. M., Kraaimaat, F. W., van Lankveld, W., Jongen, P. J. H., Jacobs, J. W. G., & Bijlsma, J. W. (2001). Beyond unfavorable thinking: The illness cognition questionnaire for chronic diseases. *Journal of Consulting and Clinical Psychology, 69*(6), 1026–1036. https://doi.org/10.1037/0022-006X.69.6.1026

Ezeh, U., Yildiz, B. O., & Azziz, R. (2013). Referral bias in defining the phenotype and prevalence of obesity in polycystic ovary syndrome. *The Journal of Clinical Endocrinology and Metabolism, 98*(6), E1088–E1096. https://doi.org/10.1210/jc.2013-1295

Fahs, B. (2011). Sex during menstruation: Race, sexual identity, and women's accounts of pleasure and disgust. *Feminism & Psychology, 21*(2), 155–178. https://doi.org/10.1177/0959353510396674

Fahs, B. (2020). *Burn it down! Feminist manifestos for the revolution*. Verso.

Fausto-Sterling, A. (2019). Gender/sex, sexual orientation, and identity are in the body: How did they get there? *Journal of Sex Research, 56*(4–5), 529–555. https://doi.org/10.1080/00224499.2019.1581883

Fife, B. L., & Wright, E. R. (2000). The dimensionality of stigma: A comparison of its impact on the self of persons with HIV/AIDS and cancer. *Journal of Health and Social Behavior, 41*(1), 50–67. https://doi.org/10.2307/2676360

Fisanick, C. (2009). Fatness (in)visible: Polycystic ovarian syndrome and the rhetoric of normative femininity. In E. Rothblum & S. Solovay (Eds.), *The fat studies reader* (pp. 106–109). New York University Press.

Fiske, S. T., Cuddy, A. J. C., Glick, P., & Xu, J. (2002). A model of (often mixed) stereotype content: Competence and warmth respectively follow from perceived status and competition. *Journal of Personality and Social Psychology, 82*(6), 878–902. https://doi.org/10.1037/0022-3514.82.6.878

Forbes, Y. N., Moffitt, R. L., Van Bokkel, M., & Donovan, C. L. (2020). Unburdening the weight of stigma: Findings from a compassion-focused group program for women with overweight and obesity. *Journal of Cognitive Psychotherapy: An International Quarterly, 34*(4), 336–357. https://doi.org/10.1891/JCPSY-D-20-00015

Fredriksen-Goldsen, K. I., Simoni, J. M., Kim, H. J., Lehavot, K., Walters, K. L., Yang, J., Hoy-Ellis, C. P., & Muraco, A. (2014). The health equity promotion model: Reconceptualization of lesbian, gay, bisexual, and transgender (LGBT) health disparities. *American Journal of Orthopsychiatry, 84*(6), 653–663. https://doi.org/10.1037/ort0000030

Frost, D. M. (2011). Social stigma and its consequences for the socially stigmatized. *Social and Personality Psychology Compass, 5*(11), 824–839. https://doi.org/10.1111/j.1751-9004.2011.00394.x

Gezer, E., Piro, B., Canturk, Z., Cetinarslan, B., Sozen, M., Selek, A., Isik, A. P., & Seal, L. J. (2021). Image satisfaction and quality of life between treatment-naïve transgender males with and without polycystic ovary syndrome. *Transgender Health*, trgh.2021.0061. Advance online publication. https://doi.org/10.1089/trgh.2021.0061

Gibbs, R. W., Jr. (2006). *Embodiment and cognitive science.* Cambridge University Press.

Gibson-Helm, M. E., Dokras, A., Karro, H., Piltonen, T., & Teede, H. J. (2018a). Knowledge and practices regarding polycystic ovary syndrome among physicians in Europe, North America, and internationally: An online questionnaire-based study. *Seminars in Reproductive Medicine, 36*(1), 19–27. https://doi.org/10.1055/s-0038-1667155

Gibson-Helm, M. E., Lucas, I. M., Boyle, J. A., & Teede, H. J. (2014). Women's experiences of polycystic ovary syndrome diagnosis. *Family Practice, 31*(5), 545–549. https://doi.org/10.1093/fampra/cmu028

Gibson-Helm, M. E., Tassone, E. C., Teede, H. J., Dokras, A., & Garad, R. (2018b). The needs of women and healthcare providers regarding polycystic ovary syndrome information, resources, and education: A systematic search and narrative review. *Seminars in Reproductive Medicine, 36*(1), 35–41. https://doi.org/10.1055/s-0038-1668086

Gibson-Helm, M. E., Teede, H., Dunaif, A., & Dokras, A. (2017). Delayed diagnosis and a lack of information associated with dissatisfaction in women with polycystic ovary syndrome. *The Journal of Clinical Endocrinology and Metabolism, 102*(2), 604–612. https://doi.org/10.1210/jc.2016-2963

Głuszak, O., Stopińska-Głuszak, U., Glinicki, P., Kapuścińska, R., Snochowska, H., Zgliczyński, W., & Dębski, R. (2012). Phenotype and metabolic disorders in polycystic ovary syndrome. *ISRN Endocrinology, 2012*, 569862. https://doi.org/10.5402/2012/569862

Goffman, E. (1963). *Stigma: Notes on the management of spoiled identity.* Prentice Hall.

Goldberg, A. E., Kuvalanka, K. A., Budge, S. L., Benz, M. B., & Smith, J. Z. (2019). Health care experiences of transgender binary and nonbinary university students. *The Counseling Psychologist, 47*(1), 59–97. https://doi.org/10.1177/0011000019827568

Gonzales, G., & Henning-Smith, C. (2017). Barriers to care among transgender and gender nonconforming adults. *The Milbank Quarterly, 95*(4), 726–748. https://doi.org/10.1111/1468-0009.12297

Gonzalez, L. O. (2000). Infertility as a transformational process: A framework for psychotherapeutic support of infertile women. *Issues in Mental Health Nursing, 21*(6), 619–633. https://doi.org/10.1080/01612840050110317

Goodman, N. F., Cobin, R. H., Futterweit, W., Glueck, J. S., Legro, R. S., Carmina, E., the American Association of Clinical Endocrinologists (AACE), the American College of Endocrinology (ACE), & the Androgen Excess and PCOS Society (AES). (2015a). American Association of Clinical Endocrinologists, American College of Endocrinology, and Androgen Excess and PCOS Society disease state clinical review: Guide to the best practices in the evaluation and treatment of polycystic ovary syndrome—Part I. *Endocrine Practice, 21*(11), 1291–1300. https://doi.org/10.4158/EP15748.DSC

Goodman, N. F., Cobin, R. H., Futterweit, W., Glueck, J. S., Legro, R. S., Carmina, E., the American Association of Clinical Endocrinologists (AACE), the American College of Endocrinology (ACE), & the Androgen Excess and PCOS Society. (2015b). American Association of Clinical Endocrinologists, American College of Endocrinology, and Androgen Excess and PCOS Society disease state clinical review: Guide to the best practices in the evaluation and treatment of polycystic ovary syndrome—Part II. *Endocrine Practice, 21*(12), 1415–1426. https://doi.org/10.4158/EP15748.DSCPT2

Govere, L., & Govere, E. M. (2016). How effective is cultural competence training of healthcare providers on improving patient satisfaction of minority groups? A systematic review of the literature. *Worldviews on Evidence-Based Nursing, 13*(6), 402–410. https://doi.org/10.1111/wvn.12176

Greenwood, E. A., Pasch, L. A., Cedars, M. I., Legro, R. S., Eisenberg, E., Huddleston, H. G., & the Eunice Kennedy Shriver National Institute of Child Health and Human Development Reproductive Medicine Network. (2018). Insulin resistance is associated with depression risk in polycystic ovary syndrome. *Fertility and Sterility, 110*(1), 27–34. https://doi.org/10.1016/j.fertnstert.2018.03.009

Greenwood, E. A., Pasch, L. A., Shinkai, K., Cedars, M. I., & Huddleston, H. G. (2019). Clinical course of depression symptoms and predictors of enduring depression risk in women with polycystic ovary syndrome: Results of a longitudinal study. *Fertility and Sterility, 111*(1), 147–156. https://doi.org/10.1016/j.fertnstert.2018.10.004

Greil, A. L. (1991). A secret stigma: The analogy between infertility and chronic illness and disability. *Advances in Medical Sociology, 2,* 17–38.

Griffiths, D. A. (2018). Shifting syndromes: Sex chromosome variations and intersex classifications. *Social Studies of Science, 48*(1), 125–148. https://doi.org/10.1177/0306312718757081

Grogan, S. (2006). Body image and health: Contemporary perspectives. *Journal of Health Psychology, 11*(4), 523–530. https://doi.org/10.1177/1359105306065013

Hahn, S., Janssen, O. E., Tan, S., Pleger, K., Mann, K., Schedlowski, M., Kimmig, R., Benson, S., Balamitsa, E., & Elsenbruch, S. (2005). Clinical and psychological correlates of quality-of-life in polycystic ovary syndrome. *European Journal of Endocrinology, 153*(6), 853–860. https://doi.org/10.1530/eje.1.02024

Hall, W. J., Chapman, M. V., Lee, K. M., Merino, Y. M., Thomas, T. W., Payne, B. K., Eng, E., Day, S. H., & Coyne-Beasley, T. (2015). Implicit racial/ethnic bias among health care professionals and its influence on health care outcomes: A systematic review. *American Journal of Public Health, 105*(12), e60–e76. https://doi.org/10.2105/AJPH.2015.302903

Hand, S. (2021). *What is medical gaslighting?* https://endometriosis.net/living/medical-gaslighting

Hart, R., & Doherty, D. A. (2015). The potential implications of a PCOS diagnosis on a woman's long-term health using data linkage. *The Journal of Clinical Endocrinology and Metabolism, 100*(3), 911–919. https://doi.org/10.1210/jc.2014-3886

Hatch, R., Rosenfield, R. L., Kim, M. H., & Tredway, D. (1981). Hirsutism: Implications, etiology, and management. *American Journal of Obstetrics and Gynecology, 140*(7), 815–830. https://doi.org/10.1016/0002-9378(81)90746-8

Hatzenbuehler, M. L. (2009). How does sexual minority stigma "get under the skin"? A psychological mediation framework. *Psychological Bulletin, 135*(5), 707–730. https://doi.org/10.1037/a0016441

Hatzenbuehler, M. L., Nolen-Hoeksema, S., & Dovidio, J. (2009). How does stigma "get under the skin"?: The mediating role of emotion regulation. *Psychological Science, 20*(10), 1282–1289. https://doi.org/10.1111/j.1467-9280.2009.02441.x

Hayfield, N., & Huxley, C. (2015). Insider and outsider perspectives: Reflections on researcher identities in research with lesbian and bisexual women. *Qualitative Research in Psychology, 12*(2), 91–106. https://doi.org/10.1080/14780887.2014.918224

Helgeson, V. S., Reynolds, K. A., & Tomich, P. L. (2006). A meta-analytic review of benefit finding and growth. *Journal of Consulting and Clinical Psychology, 74*(5), 797–816. https://doi.org/10.1037/0022-006X.74.5.797

Himelein, M. J., & Thatcher, S. S. (2006a). Depression and body image among women with polycystic ovary syndrome. *Journal of Health Psychology, 11*(4), 613–625. https://doi.org/10.1177/1359105306065021

Himelein, M. J., & Thatcher, S. S. (2006b). Polycystic ovary syndrome and mental health: A review. *Obstetrical & Gynecological Survey, 61*(11), 723–732. https://doi.org/10.1097/01.ogx.0000243772.33357.84

Hoeger, K. M., Dokras, A., & Piltonen, T. (2021). Update on PCOS: Consequences, challenges, and guiding treatment. *The Journal of Clinical Endocrinology and Metabolism, 106*(3), e1071–e1083. https://doi.org/10.1210/clinem/dgaa839

House, J. S., Umberson, D., & Landis, K. R. (1988). Structures and processes of social support. *Annual Review of Sociology, 14*(1), 293–318. https://doi.org/10.1146/annurev.so.14.080188.001453

Hung, J. H., Hu, L. Y., Tsai, S. J., Yang, A. C., Huang, M. W., Chen, P. M., Wang, S. L., Lu, T., & Shen, C. C. (2014). Risk of psychiatric disorders following polycystic ovary syndrome: A nationwide population-based cohort study. *PLOS ONE, 9*(5), e97041. https://doi.org/10.1371/journal.pone.0097041

Hunger, J. M., Major, B., Blodorn, A., & Miller, C. T. (2015). Weighed down by stigma: How weight-based social identity threat contributes to weight gain and poor health. *Social and Personality Psychology Compass, 9*(6), 255–268. https://doi.org/10.1111/spc3.12172

Hyde, J. S., Bigler, R. S., Joel, D., Tate, C. C., & van Anders, S. M. (2019). The future of sex and gender in psychology: Five challenges to the gender binary. *American Psychologist, 74*(2), 171–193. https://doi.org/10.1037/amp0000307

Institute of Medicine. (2003). *Unequal treatment: Confronting racial and ethnic disparities in health care*. The National Academies Press.

Jason, J. (2011). Polycystic ovary syndrome in the United States: Clinical visit rates, characteristics, and associated health care costs. *Archives of Internal Medicine, 171*(13), 1209–1211. https://doi.org/10.1001/archinternmed.2011.288

Jímenez-Loaisa, A., Beltran-Carrillo, V. J., Gonzalez-Cutre, D., & Jennings, G. (2020). Healthism and the experiences of social, healthcare and self-stigma of women with higher-weight. *Social Theory & Health, 18*(4), 410–424. https://doi.org/10.1057/s41285-019-00118-9

Johnston-Robledo, I., & Chrisler, J. C. (2013). The menstrual mark: Menstruation as social stigma. *Sex Roles, 68*(1–2), 9–18. https://doi.org/10.1007/s11199-011-0052-z

Jones, E. E., Farina, A., Hastorf, A. H., Markus, H., Miller, D. T., & Scott, R. A. (1984). *Social stigma: The psychology of marked relationships*. W. H. Freeman.

Jones, G. L., Hall, J. M., Lashen, H. L., Balen, A. H., & Ledger, W. L. (2011). Health-related quality of life among adolescents with polycystic ovary syndrome. *Journal of Obstetric, Gynecologic, and Neonatal Nursing, 40*(5), 577–588. https://doi.org/10.1111/j.1552-6909.2011.01279.x

Jowett, A., & Peel, E. (2009). Chronic illness in non-heterosexual contexts: An online survey of experiences. *Feminism & Psychology, 19*(4), 454–474. https://doi.org/10.1177/0959353509342770

Kattari, S. K., Curley, K. M., Bakko, M., & Misiolek, B. A. (2020). Development and validation of the trans-inclusive provider scale. *American Journal of Preventive Medicine, 58*(5), 707–714. https://doi.org/10.1016/j.amepre.2019.12.005

Katz, R. C., Flasher, L., Cacciapaglia, H., & Nelson, S. (2001). The psychosocial impact of cancer and lupus: A cross validation study that extends the generality of "benefit-finding" in patients with chronic disease. *Journal of Behavioral Medicine, 24*(6), 561–571. https://doi.org/10.1023/A:1012939310459

Keegan, A., Liao, L. M., & Boyle, M. (2003). "Hirsutism": A psychological analysis. *Journal of Health Psychology, 8*(3), 327–345. https://doi.org/10.1177/13591053030083004

Kennedy, J. (2019). *PCOS: The new science of completely reversing symptoms while restoring hormone balance, mental health, and fertility for good.* Independently Published.

Kessler, R. C., Chiu, W. T., Demler, O., Merikangas, K. R., & Walters, E. E. (2005). Prevalence, severity, and comorbidity of 12-month *DSM-IV* disorders in the National Comorbidity Survey Replication. *Archives of General Psychiatry, 62*(6), 617–627. https://doi.org/10.1001/archpsyc.62.6.617

Khomami, M. B., Joham, A. E., Boyle, J. A., Piltonen, T., Silagy, M., Arora, C., Misso, M. L., Teede, H. J., & Moran, L. J. (2019). Increased maternal pregnancy complications in polycystic ovary syndrome appear to be independent of obesity—A systematic review, meta-analysis, and meta-regression. *Obesity Reviews, 20*(5), 659–674. https://doi.org/10.1111/obr.12829

Khomami, M. B., Tehrani, F. R., Hashemi, S., Farahmand, M., & Azizi, F. (2015). Of PCOS symptoms, hirsutism has the most significant impact on the quality of life of Iranian women. *PLOS ONE, 10*(4), e0123608. https://doi.org/10.1371/journal.pone.0123608

Kissling, E. A. (1996). Bleeding out loud: Communication about menstruation. *Feminism & Psychology, 6*(4), 481–504. https://doi.org/10.1177/0959353596064002

Kitzinger, C., & Willmott, J. (2002). "The thief of womanhood": Women's experience of polycystic ovarian syndrome. *Social Science & Medicine, 54*(3), 349–361. https://doi.org/10.1016/S0277-9536(01)00034-X

Knochenhauer, E. S., Key, T. J., Kahsar-Miller, M., Waggoner, W., Boots, L. R., & Azziz, R. (1998). Prevalence of the polycystic ovary syndrome in unselected black and white women of the southeastern United States: A prospective study. *The Journal of Clinical Endocrinology and Metabolism, 83*(9), 3078–3082. https://doi.org/10.1210/jc.83.9.3078

Kogure, G. S., Ribeiro, V. B., Lopes, I. P., Furtado, C. L. M., Kodato, S., Silva de Sá, M. F., Ferriani, R. A., Lara, L. A. D. S., & Maria Dos Reis, R. (2019). Body image and its relationships with sexual functioning, anxiety, and depression in women with polycystic ovary syndrome. *Journal of Affective Disorders, 253,* 385–393. https://doi.org/10.1016/j.jad.2019.05.006

Kowalczyk, R., Skrzypulec, V., Lew-Starowicz, Z., Nowosielski, K., Grabski, B., & Merk, W. (2012). Psychological gender of patients with polycystic ovary

Kattari, S. K., Curley, K. M., Bakko, M., & Misiolek, B. A. (2020). Development and validation of the trans-inclusive provider scale. *American Journal of Preventive Medicine, 58*(5), 707–714. https://doi.org/10.1016/j.amepre.2019.12.005

Katz, R. C., Flasher, L., Cacciapaglia, H., & Nelson, S. (2001). The psychosocial impact of cancer and lupus: A cross validation study that extends the generality of "benefit-finding" in patients with chronic disease. *Journal of Behavioral Medicine, 24*(6), 561–571. https://doi.org/10.1023/A:1012939310459

Keegan, A., Liao, L. M., & Boyle, M. (2003). "Hirsutism": A psychological analysis. *Journal of Health Psychology, 8*(3), 327–345. https://doi.org/10.1177/13591053030083004

Kennedy, J. (2019). *PCOS: The new science of completely reversing symptoms while restoring hormone balance, mental health, and fertility for good.* Independently Published.

Kessler, R. C., Chiu, W. T., Demler, O., Merikangas, K. R., & Walters, E. E. (2005). Prevalence, severity, and comorbidity of 12-month *DSM-IV* disorders in the National Comorbidity Survey Replication. *Archives of General Psychiatry, 62*(6), 617–627. https://doi.org/10.1001/archpsyc.62.6.617

Khomami, M. B., Joham, A. E., Boyle, J. A., Piltonen, T., Silagy, M., Arora, C., Misso, M. L., Teede, H. J., & Moran, L. J. (2019). Increased maternal pregnancy complications in polycystic ovary syndrome appear to be independent of obesity—A systematic review, meta-analysis, and meta-regression. *Obesity Reviews, 20*(5), 659–674. https://doi.org/10.1111/obr.12829

Khomami, M. B., Tehrani, F. R., Hashemi, S., Farahmand, M., & Azizi, F. (2015). Of PCOS symptoms, hirsutism has the most significant impact on the quality of life of Iranian women. *PLOS ONE, 10*(4), e0123608. https://doi.org/10.1371/journal.pone.0123608

Kissling, E. A. (1996). Bleeding out loud: Communication about menstruation. *Feminism & Psychology, 6*(4), 481–504. https://doi.org/10.1177/0959353596064002

Kitzinger, C., & Willmott, J. (2002). "The thief of womanhood": Women's experience of polycystic ovarian syndrome. *Social Science & Medicine, 54*(3), 349–361. https://doi.org/10.1016/S0277-9536(01)00034-X

Knochenhauer, E. S., Key, T. J., Kahsar-Miller, M., Waggoner, W., Boots, L. R., & Azziz, R. (1998). Prevalence of the polycystic ovary syndrome in unselected Black and White women of the southeastern United States: A prospective study. *The Journal of Clinical Endocrinology and Metabolism, 83*(9), 3078–3082. https://doi.org/10.1210/jc.83.9.3078

Kogure, G. S., Ribeiro, V. B., Lopes, I. P., Furtado, C. L. M., Kodato, S., Silva de Sá, M. F., Ferriani, R. A., Lara, L. A. D. S., & Maria Dos Reis, R. (2019). Body image and its relationships with sexual functioning, anxiety, and depression in women with polycystic ovary syndrome. *Journal of Affective Disorders, 253*, 385–393. https://doi.org/10.1016/j.jad.2019.05.006

Kowalczyk, R., Skrzypulec, V., Lew-Starowicz, Z., Nowosielski, K., Grabski, B., & Merk, W. (2012). Psychological gender of patients with polycystic ovary

Li, Y., Li, Y., Yu Ng, E. H., Stener-Victorin, E., Hou, L., Wu, T., Han, F., & Wu, X. (2011). Polycystic ovary syndrome is associated with negatively variable impacts on domains of health-related quality of life: Evidence from a meta-analysis. *Fertility and Sterility, 96*(2), 452–458. https://doi.org/10.1016/j.fertnstert.2011.05.072

Lim, S. S., Davies, M. J., Norman, R. J., & Moran, L. J. (2012). Overweight, obesity and central obesity in women with polycystic ovary syndrome: A systematic review and meta-analysis. *Human Reproduction Update, 18*(6), 618–637. https://doi.org/10.1093/humupd/dms030

Lim, S. S., Kakoly, N. S., Tan, J. W. J., Fitzgerald, G., Bahri Khomami, M., Joham, A. E., Cooray, S. D., Misso, M. L., Norman, R. J., Harrison, C. L., Ranasinha, S., Teede, H. J., & Moran, L. J. (2019). Metabolic syndrome in polycystic ovary syndrome: A systematic review, meta-analysis and meta-regression. *Obesity Reviews, 20*(2), 339–352. https://doi.org/10.1111/obr.12762

Lin, A. W., Bergomi, E. J., Dollahite, J. S., Sobal, J., Hoeger, K. M., & Lujan, M. E. (2018). Trust in physicians and medical experience differ between women with and without polycystic ovary syndrome. *Journal of the Endocrine Society, 2*(9), 1001–1009. https://doi.org/10.1210/js.2018-00181

Link, B. G., Cullen, F. T., Struening, E., Shrout, P. E., & Dohrenwend, B. P. (1989). A modified labeling theory approach to mental disorders: An empirical assessment. *American Sociological Review, 54*(3), 400–423. https://doi.org/10.2307/2095613

Link, B. G., & Phelan, J. C. (2001). Conceptualizing stigma. *Annual Review of Sociology, 27*(1), 363–385. https://doi.org/10.1146/annurev.soc.27.1.363

Liu, M., Murthi, S., & Poretsky, L. (2020). Polycystic ovary syndrome and gender identity. *The Yale Journal of Biology and Medicine, 93*(4), 529–537.

Lizneva, D., Suturina, L., Walker, W., Brakta, S., Gavrilova-Jordan, L., & Azziz, R. (2016). Criteria, prevalence, and phenotypes of polycystic ovary syndrome. *Fertility and Sterility, 106*(1), 6–15. https://doi.org/10.1016/j.fertnstert.2016.05.003

Lobo, R. A. (1995). A disorder without identity: "HCA," "PCO," "PCOD," "PCOS," "SLS." What are we to call it?! *Fertility and Sterility, 63*(6), 1158–1160. https://doi.org/10.1016/S0015-0282(16)57589-X

Lorde, A. (1984). *Sister outsider*. Crossing Press.

Macy, J. (2007). *World as lover, world as self*. Parallax Press.

Major, B., Dovidio, J. F., Link, B. G., & Calabrese, S. K. (2018). Stigma and its implications for health: Introduction and overview. In B. Major, J. F. Dovidio, & B. G. Link (Eds.), *The Oxford handbook of stigma, discrimination, and health* (pp. 3–28). Oxford University Press.

Major, B., Eliezer, D., & Rieck, H. (2012). The psychological weight of weight stigma. *Social Psychological & Personality Science, 3*(6), 651–658. https://doi.org/10.1177/1948550611434400

Major, B., Mendes, W. B., & Dovidio, J. F. (2013). Intergroup relations and health disparities: A social psychological perspective. *Health Psychology, 32*(5), 514–524. https://doi.org/10.1037/a0030358

Major, B., & O'Brien, L. T. (2005). The social psychology of stigma. *Annual Review of Psychology, 56*(1), 393–421. https://doi.org/10.1146/annurev.psych. 56.091103.070137

Major, B., Tomiyama, A. J., & Hunger, J. M. (2018). The negative and bidirectional effects of weight stigma on health. In B. Major, J. F. Dovidio, & B. G. Link (Eds.), *The Oxford handbook of stigma, discrimination, and health* (pp. 499–519). Oxford University Press.

Malatino, H. (2019). *Queer embodiment: Monstrosity, medical violence, and intersex experience.* University of Nebraska Press. https://doi.org/10.2307/j.ctvckq9pv

Malik-Aslam, A., Reaney, M. D., & Speight, J. (2010). The suitability of polycystic ovary syndrome-specific questionnaires for measuring the impact of PCOS on quality of life in clinical trials. *Value in Health, 13*(4), 440–446. https:// doi.org/10.1111/j.1524-4733.2010.00696.x

March, W. A., Moore, V. M., Willson, K. J., Phillips, D. I. W., Norman, R. J., & Davies, M. J. (2010). The prevalence of polycystic ovary syndrome in a community sample assessed under contrasting diagnostic criteria. *Human Reproduction, 25*(2), 544–551. https://doi.org/10.1093/humrep/dep399

Marrow, A. J. (1969). *The practical theorist: The life and work of Kurt Lewin.* Basic Books.

Martin, M. L., Halling, K., Eek, D., Krohe, M., & Paty, J. (2017). Understanding polycystic ovary syndrome from the patient perspective: A concept elicitation patient interview study. *Health and Quality of Life Outcomes, 15*(1), 162–172. https://doi.org/10.1186/s12955-017-0736-3

Martz, E., & Livneh, H. (2016). Psychosocial adaptation to disability within the context of positive psychology: Findings from the literature. *Journal of Occupational Rehabilitation, 26*(1), 4–12. https://doi.org/10.1007/s10926-015-9598-x

McCook, J. G., Bailey, B. A., Williams, S. L., Anand, S., & Reame, N. E. (2015). Differential contribution of polycystic ovary syndrome (PCOS) manifestations to psychological symptoms. *The Journal of Behavioral Health Services & Research, 42*(3), 383–394. https://doi.org/10.1007/s11414-013-9382-7

Merleau-Ponty, M. (1962). *Phenomenology of perception.* Routledge.

Meyer, I. H. (2013). Prejudice, social stress, and mental health in lesbian, gay, and bisexual populations: Conceptual issues and research evidence. *Psychology of Sexual Orientation and Gender Diversity, 1*(Suppl.), 3–26. https://doi.org/ 10.1037/2329-0382.1.S.3

Michelmore, K. F., Balen, A. H., Dunger, D. B., & Vessey, M. P. (1999). Polycystic ovaries and associated clinical and biochemical features in young women. *Clinical Endocrinology, 51*(6), 779–786. https://doi.org/10.1046/j.1365-2265. 1999.00886.x

Millin, P. T. (2009). *Women, writing, and soul-making: Creativity and the sacred feminine.* Story Water Press.

Mohr, D. C., Dick, L. P., Russo, D., Pinn, J., Boudewyn, A. C., Likosky, W., & Goodkin, D. E. (1999). The psychosocial impact of multiple sclerosis: Exploring the patient's perspective. *Health Psychology, 18*(4), 376–382. https://doi.org/10.1037/0278-6133.18.4.376

Mondragón-Ceballos, R., García Granados, M. D., Cerda-Molina, A. L., Chavira-Ramírez, R., & Hernández-López, L. E. (2015). Waist-to-hip ratio, but not body mass index, is associated with testosterone and estradiol concentrations in young women. *International Journal of Endocrinology, 2015*, 654046. https://doi.org/10.1155/2015/654046

Moradi, F., Ghadiri-Anari, A., Dehghani, A., Reza Vaziri, S., & Enjezab, B. (2020). The effectiveness of counseling based on acceptance and commitment therapy on body image and self-esteem in polycystic ovary syndrome: An RCT. *International Journal of Reproductive Biomedicine, 18*(4), 243–252. https://doi.org/10.18502/ijrm.v13i4.6887

Morotti, E., Persico, N., Battaglia, B., Fabbri, R., Meriggiola, M. C., Venturoli, S., & Battaglia, C. (2013). Body imaging and sexual behavior in lean women with polycystic ovary syndrome. *Journal of Sexual Medicine, 10*(11), 2752–2760. https://doi.org/10.1111/jsm.12284

National Academies of Science, Engineering, and Medicine. (2017). *Communities in action: Pathways to health equity.* The National Academies Press.

National Institutes of Health. (n.d.). *Evidence-based methodology workshop on polycystic ovary syndrome.* https://prevention.nih.gov/research-priorities/research-needs-and-gaps/pathways-prevention/evidence-based-methodology-workshop-polycystic-ovary-syndrome-pcos

Naz, M. S. G., Tehrani, F. R., Ahmadi, F., Alavi Majd, H., & Ozgoli, G. (2019). Threats to feminine identity as the main concern of Iranian adolescents with polycystic ovary syndrome: A qualitative study. *Journal of Pediatric Nursing, 49*, e42–e47. https://doi.org/10.1016/j.pedn.2019.08.010

Neff, K. (2003). Self-compassion: An alternative conceptualization of a healthy attitude toward oneself. *Self and Identity, 2*(2), 85–101. https://doi.org/10.1080/15298860309032

O'Hara, L., Ahmed, H., & Elashie, S. (2021). Evaluating the impact of a brief Health at Every Size®-informed health promotion activity on body positivity and internalized weight-based oppression. *Body Image, 37*, 225–237. https://doi.org/10.1016/j.bodyim.2021.02.006

Pachankis, J. E. (2007). The psychological implications of concealing a stigma: A cognitive-affective-behavioral model. *Psychological Bulletin, 133*(2), 328–345. https://doi.org/10.1037/0033-2909.133.2.328

Palmer, P. (1999). *Let your life speak: Listening for the voice of vocation.* Jossey-Bass.

Papadopoulos, S., & Brennan, L. (2015). Correlates of weight stigma in adults with overweight and obesity: A systematic literature review. *Obesity, 23*(9), 1743–1760. https://doi.org/10.1002/oby.21187

Paradies, Y., Truong, M., & Priest, N. (2014). A systematic review of the extent and measurement of healthcare provider racism. *Journal of General Internal Medicine, 29*(2), 364–387. https://doi.org/10.1007/s11606-013-2583-1

Park, C. L. (2009). Overview of theoretical perspectives. In C. L. Park, S. C. Lechner, M. H. Antoni, & A. L. Stanton (Eds.), *Medical illness and positive life change: Can crisis lead to personal transformation?* (pp. 11–30). American Psychological Association. https://doi.org/10.1037/11854-001

Park, C. L. (2010). Making sense of the meaning literature: An integrative review of meaning making and its effects on adjustment to stressful life events. *Psychological Bulletin, 136*(2), 257–301. https://doi.org/10.1037/a0018301

Park, C. L. (2013). Spirituality and meaning making in cancer survivorship. In K. D. Markman, T. Proulx, & M. J. Lindberg (Eds.), *The psychology of meaning* (pp. 257–277). American Psychological Association. https://doi.org/10.1037/14040-013

Parker, M., Warren, A., Nair, S., & Barnard, M. (2020). Adherence to treatment for polycystic ovarian syndrome: A systematic review. *PLOS ONE, 15*(2), e0228586. https://doi.org/10.1371/journal.pone.0228586

Penner, L., Phelan, S. M., Earnshaw, V., Albrecht, T. L., & Dovidio, J. F. (2018). Patient stigma, medical interactions, and health care disparities: A selective review. In B. Major, J. F. Dovidio, & B. G. Link (Eds.), *The Oxford handbook of stigma, discrimination, and health* (pp. 183–201). Oxford University Press.

Perez, C. C. (2019). *Invisible women: Data bias in a world designed for men.* Abrams Press.

Pescosolido, B. A., & Martin, J. K. (2015). The stigma complex. *Annual Review of Sociology, 41*(1), 87–116. https://doi.org/10.1146/annurev-soc-071312-145702

Peters, M. F., & Massey, G. (1983). Mundane extreme environmental stress in family stress theories: The case of Black families in White America. *Marriage & Family Review, 6*(1–2), 193–218. https://doi.org/10.1300/J002v06n01_10

Pfister, G., & Rømer, K. (2017). "It's not very feminine to have a mustache": Experiences of Danish women with polycystic ovary syndrome. *Health Care for Women International, 38*(2), 167–186. https://doi.org/10.1080/07399332.2016.1236108

Polson, D. W., Adams, J., Wadsworth, J., & Franks, S. (1988). Polycystic ovaries—A common finding in normal women. *The Lancet, 1*(8590), 870–872. https://doi.org/10.1016/S0140-6736(88)91612-1

Poteat, T. C., & Singh, A. A. (2017). Conceptualizing trauma in clinical settings: Iatrogenic harm and bias. In K. L. Eckstrand & J. Potter (Eds.), *Trauma, resilience, and health promotion in LGBT patients: What every healthcare provider should know* (pp. 25–33). Springer. https://doi.org/10.1007/978-3-319-54509-7_3

Pounders, K., & Mason, M. (2018). Embodiment, illness, and gender: The intersected and disrupted identities of young women with breast cancer. *Consumer Culture Theory, 19*, 111–122. https://doi.org/10.1108/S0885-211120180000019007

Puhl, R. M., & Brownell, K. D. (2001). Bias, discrimination, and obesity. *Obesity Research, 9*(12), 788–805. https://doi.org/10.1038/oby.2001.108

Puhl, R. M., & Heuer, C. A. (2009). The stigma of obesity: A review and update. *Obesity, 17*(5), 941–964. https://doi.org/10.1038/oby.2008.636

Puhl, R. M., & Latner, J. D. (2007). Stigma, obesity, and the health of the nation's children. *Psychological Bulletin, 133*(4), 557–580. https://doi.org/10.1037/0033-2909.133.4.557

Puhl, R. M., Moss-Racusin, C. A., Schwartz, M. B., & Brownell, K. D. (2008). Weight stigmatization and bias reduction: Perspectives of overweight and obese adults. *Health Education Research, 23*(2), 347–358. https://doi.org/10.1093/her/cym052

Purdie-Vaughns, V., & Eibach, R. P. (2008). Intersectional invisibility: The distinctive advantages and disadvantages of multiple subordinate-group identities. *Sex Roles, 59*(5–6), 377–391. https://doi.org/10.1007/s11199-008-9424-4

QSR International. (2015). *NVivo* (Version 11). https://www.qsrinternational.com/nvivo-qualitative-data-analysis-software/home

Rahimi-Ardabili, H., Reynolds, R., Vartanian, L. R., McLeod, L. V. D., & Zwar, N. (2018). A systematic review of the efficacy of interventions that aim to increase self-compassion on nutrition habits, eating behaviours, body weight and body image. *Mindfulness, 9*(2), 388–400. https://doi.org/10.1007/s12671-017-0804-0

Raja, S., Hasnain, M., Hoersch, M., Gove-Yin, S., & Rajagopalan, C. (2015). Trauma informed care in medicine: Current knowledge and future research directions. *Family & Community Health, 38*(3), 216–226. https://doi.org/10.1097/FCH.0000000000000071

Rajesh, R., Tampi, R., & Balachandran, S. (2019). The case for behavioral health integration into primary care. *The Journal of Family Practice, 68*(5), 278–284.

Rand, K., Vallis, M., Aston, M., Price, S., Piccinini-Vallis, H., Rehman, L., & Kirk, S. F. L. (2017). "It is not the diet; it is the mental part we need help with." A multilevel analysis of psychological, emotional, and social well-being in obesity. *International Journal of Qualitative Studies on Health and Well-Being, 12*(1), 1306421. https://doi.org/10.1080/17482631.2017.1306421

Richards, R. (2019). Shame, silence and resistance: How my narratives of academia and kidney disease entwine. *Feminism & Psychology, 29*(2), 269–285. https://doi.org/10.1177/0959353518786757

Ridenour, A. F., Yorgason, J. B., & Peterson, B. (2009). The infertility resilience model: Assessing individuals, couple, and external predictive factors. *Contemporary Family Therapy, 31*(1), 34–51. https://doi.org/10.1007/s10591-008-9077-z

Riestenberg, C., Jagasia, A., Markovic, D., Buyalos, R. P., & Azziz, R. (2022). Health care-related economic burden of polycystic syndrome in the United States: Pregnancy-related and long-term health consequences. *The Journal of Clinical Endocrinology and Metabolism, 107*(2), 575–585. https://doi.org/10.1210/clinem/dgab613

Roberts, K., Dowell, A., & Nie, J. B. (2019). Attempting rigour and replicability in thematic analysis of qualitative research data; a case study of codebook development. *BMC Medical Research Methodology, 19*(1), 66. https://doi.org/10.1186/s12874-019-0707-y

Rodriguez-Paris, D., Remlinger-Molenda, A., Kurzawa, R., Głowińska, A., Spaczyński, R., Rybakowski, F., Pawełczyk, L., & Banaszewska, B. (2019). Występowanie zaburzeń psychicznych u kobiet z zespołem policystycznych jajników [Psychiatric disorders in women with polycystic ovary syndrome]. *Psychiatria Polska, 53*(4), 955–966. https://doi.org/10.12740/PP/OnlineFirst/93105

Rodriguez-Seijas, C., Burton, C. L., Adeyinka, O., & Pachankis, J. E. (2019). On the quantitative study of multiple marginalization: Paradox and potential solution. *Stigma and Health, 4*(4), 495–502. https://doi.org/10.1037/sah0000166

Russo, N. P. (1976). The motherhood mandate. *Journal of Social Issues, 32*(3), 143–153. https://doi.org/10.1111/j.1540-4560.1976.tb02603.x

Samardzic, T., Soucie, K., Schramer, K., & Katzman, R. (2021). "I didn't feel normal": Young Canadian women's experiences with polycystic ovary syndrome. *Feminism & Psychology, 31*(4), 571–590. https://doi.org/10.1177/09593535211030748

Sanchez, N. (2018). Suitability of the National Health Care surveys to examine behavioral health services associated with polycystic ovary syndrome. *The Journal of Behavioral Health Services & Research, 45*(2), 252–268. https://doi.org/10.1007/s11414-016-9543-6

Schwarzer, R., & Leppin, A. (1991). Social support and health: A theoretical and empirical overview. *Journal of Social and Personal Relationships, 8*(1), 99–127. https://doi.org/10.1177/0265407591081005

Serano, J. (2016). *Whipping girl: A transsexual woman on sexism and the scapegoating of femininity.* Seal Press.

Shelton, J. N., Richeson, J. A., & Salvatore, J. (2005). Expecting to be the target of prejudice: Implications for interethnic interactions. *Personality and Social Psychology Bulletin, 31*(9), 1189–1202. https://doi.org/10.1177/0146167205274894

Shroff, R., Syrop, C. H., Davis, W., Van Voorhis, B. J., & Dokras, A. (2007). Risk of metabolic complications in the new PCOS phenotypes based on the Rotterdam criteria. *Fertility and Sterility, 88*(5), 1389–1395. https://doi.org/10.1016/j.fertnstert.2007.01.032

Sikorski, C., Luppa, M., Luck, T., & Riedel-Heller, S. G. (2015). Weight stigma "gets under the skin"—Evidence for an adapted psychological mediation framework: A systematic review. *Obesity, 23*(2), 266–276. https://doi.org/10.1002/oby.20952

Sills, E. S., Perloe, M., Tucker, M. J., Kaplan, C. R., Genton, M. G., & Schattman, G. L. (2001). Diagnostic and treatment characteristics of polycystic ovary syndrome: Descriptive measurements of patient perception and awareness from 657 confidential self-reports. *BMC Women's Health, 1*(1), 3. https://doi.org/10.1186/1472-6874-1-3

Snyder, B. S. (2006). The lived experience of women diagnosed with polycystic ovary syndrome. *Journal of Obstetric, Gynecologic, and Neonatal Nursing, 35*(3), 385–392. https://doi.org/10.1111/j.1552-6909.2006.00047.x

Solar, O., & Irwin, A. (2010). *A conceptual framework for action on the social determinants of health: Social determinants of health discussion paper 2 (Policy and Practice)*. World Health Organization.

Soucie, K., Samardzic, T., Schramer, K., Ly, C., & Katzman, R. (2021). The diagnostic experiences of women with polycystic ovary syndrome (PCOS) in Ontario, Canada. *Qualitative Health Research, 31*(3), 523–534. https://doi.org/10.1177/1049732320971235

Spencer, A. L., Bost, J. E., & McNeil, M. (2007). Do women's health internal medicine residency tracks make a difference? *Journal of Women's Health, 16*(8), 1219–1223. https://doi.org/10.1089/jwh.2006.0274

Stangl, A. L., Earnshaw, V. A., Logie, C. H., van Brakel, W., C Simbayi, L., Barré, I., & Dovidio, J. F. (2019). The Health Stigma and Discrimination Framework: A global, crosscutting framework to inform research, intervention development, and policy on health-related stigmas. *BMC Medicine, 17*(1), 31. https://doi.org/10.1186/s12916-019-1271-3

Stanton, A. L., Lobel, M., Sears, S., & DeLuca, R. S. (2002). Psychosocial aspects of selected issues in women's reproductive health: Current status and future directions. *Journal of Consulting and Clinical Psychology, 70*(3), 751–770. https://doi.org/10.1037/0022-006X.70.3.751

Stefanaki, C., Bacopoulou, F., Livadas, S., Kandaraki, A., Karachalios, A., Chrousos, G. P., & Diamanti-Kandarakis, E. (2015). Impact of a mindfulness stress management program on stress, anxiety, depression and quality of life in women with polycystic ovary syndrome: A randomized controlled trial. *Stress, 18*(1), 57–66. https://doi.org/10.3109/10253890.2014.974030

Stein, I. F., & Leventhal, M. L. (1935). Amenorrhea associated with bilateral polycystic ovaries. *American Journal of Obstetrics and Gynecology, 29*(2), 181–191. https://doi.org/10.1016/S0002-9378(15)30642-6

Stovall, D. W., Scriver, J. L., Clayton, A. H., Williams, C. D., & Pastore, L. M. (2012). Sexual function in women with polycystic ovary syndrome. *Journal of Sexual Medicine, 9*(1), 224–230. https://doi.org/10.1111/j.1743-6109.2011.02539.x

Strayed, C. (2012). *Tiny beautiful things: Advice on love and life from Dear Sugar*. Vintage.

Substance Abuse and Mental Health Services Administration. (2014). *SAMHSA's concept of trauma and guidance for a trauma-informed approach* (HHS Publication No. SMA 14-4884).

Tavris, C. (1992). *The mismeasure of woman*. Simon & Schuster.

Tay, C. T., Teede, H. J., Loxton, D., Kulkarni, J., & Joham, A. E. (2020). Psychiatric comorbidities and adverse childhood experiences in women with self-reported polycystic ovary syndrome: An Australian population-based study. *Psychoneuroendocrinology, 116*, 104678. https://doi.org/10.1016/j.psyneuen.2020.104678

Tedeschi, R. G., & Calhoun, L. G. (1996). The Posttraumatic Growth Inventory: Measuring the positive legacy of trauma. *Journal of Traumatic Stress, 9*(3), 455–471. https://doi.org/10.1002/jts.2490090305

Tedeschi, R. G., & Calhoun, L. G. (2012). Pathways to personal transformation: Theoretical and empirical developments. In P. T. P. Wong (Ed.), *The human quest for meaning* (pp. 559–572). Routledge.

Tedeschi, R. G., & Calhoun, L. G. (2014). *Handbook of posttraumatic growth.* Routledge.

Teede, H., Deeks, A., & Moran, L. (2010). Polycystic ovary syndrome: A complex condition with psychological, reproductive and metabolic manifestations that impacts on health across the lifespan. *BMC Medicine, 8*(1), 41–51. https://doi.org/10.1186/1741-7015-8-41

Teede, H. J., Misso, M. L., Costello, M. F., Dokras, A., Laven, J., Moran, L., Piltonen, T., Norman, R. J., Andersen, M., Azziz, R., Balen, A., Baye, E., Boyle, J., Brennan, L., Broekmans, F., Dabadghao, P., Devoto, L., Dewailly, D., Downes, L., . . . Yildiz, B. O., & the International PCOS Network. (2018). Recommendations from the international evidence-based guideline for the assessment and management of polycystic ovary syndrome. *Human Reproduction, 33*(9), 1602–1618. https://doi.org/10.1093/humrep/dey256

Teede, H. J., Misso, M. L., Deeks, A. A., Moran, L. J., Stuckey, B. G., Wong, J. L., Norman, R. J., Costello, M. F., & the Guideline Development Groups. (2011). Assessment and management of polycystic ovary syndrome: Summary of an evidence-based guideline. *The Medical Journal of Australia, 195*(6), S65–S112. https://doi.org/10.5694/mja11.10915

Thatcher, S. S. (2000). *Polycystic ovary syndrome: The hidden epidemic.* Perspectives Press.

Thorpe, C., Arbeau, K. J., & Budlong, B. (2019). "I drew the parts of my body in proportion to how much PCOS ruined them": Experiences of polycystic ovary syndrome through drawings. *Health Psychology Open, 6*(2), 2055102919896238. https://doi.org/10.1177/2055102919896238

Toerien, M., & Wilkinson, S. (2003). Gender and body hair: Constructing the feminine woman. *Women's Studies International Forum, 26*(4), 333–344. https://doi.org/10.1016/S0277-5395(03)00078-5

Toerien, M., & Wilkinson, S. (2004). Exploring the depilation norm: A qualitative questionnaire study of women's body hair removal. *Qualitative Research in Psychology, 1*, 69–92.

Toerien, M., Wilkinson, S., & Choi, P. Y. L. (2005). Body hair removal: The "mundane" production of normative femininity. *Sex Roles, 52*(5–6), 399–406. https://doi.org/10.1007/s11199-005-2682-5

Tomlinson, J., Pinkney, J., Adams, L., Stenhouse, E., Bendall, A., Corrigan, O., & Letherby, G. (2017). The diagnosis and lived experience of polycystic ovary syndrome: A qualitative study. *Journal of Advanced Nursing, 73*(10), 2318–2326. https://doi.org/10.1111/jan.13300

Toosy, S., Sodi, R., & Pappachan, J. M. (2018). Lean polycystic ovary syndrome (PCOS): An evidence-based practical approach. *Journal of Diabetes and Metabolic Disorders, 17*(2), 277–285. https://doi.org/10.1007/s40200-018-0371-5

Tzalazidis, R., & Oinonen, K. A. (2021). Continuum of symptoms in poly-cystic ovary syndrome (PCOS): Links with sexual behavior and unrestricted sociosexuality. *Journal of Sex Research, 58*(4), 532–544. https://doi.org/10.1080/00224499.2020.1726273

Umberson, D. (1987). Family status and health behaviors: Social control as a dimension of social integration. *Journal of Health and Social Behavior, 28*(3), 306–319. https://doi.org/10.2307/2136848

U.S. Department of Health and Human Services, Office of Disease Prevention and Health Promotion. (n.d.). *Healthy People 2030.* https://health.gov/healthypeople/objectives-and-data/social-determinants-health

Ussher, J. C. C., & Perz, J. (Eds.). (2019). *Routledge international handbook of women's sexual and reproductive health.* Routledge. https://doi.org/10.4324/9781351035620

Vaismoradi, M., Jones, J., Turunen, H., & Snelgrove, S. (2016). Theme development in qualitative content analysis and thematic analysis. *Journal of Nursing Education and Practice, 6*(5), 100–110. https://doi.org/10.5430/jnep.v6n5p100

van Anders, S. M. (2015). Beyond sexual orientation: Integrating gender/sex and diverse sexualities via sexual configurations theory. *Archives of Sexual Behavior, 44*(5), 1177–1213. https://doi.org/10.1007/s10508-015-0490-8

van Anders, S. M., & Hampson, E. (2005). Waist-to-hip ratio is positively associated with bioavailable testosterone but negatively associated with sexual desire in healthy premenopausal women. *Psychosomatic Medicine, 67*(2), 246–250. https://doi.org/10.1097/01.psy.0000151747.22904.d7

Veltman-Verhulst, S. M., Boivin, J., Eijkemans, M. J. C., & Fauser, B. J. C. M. (2012). Emotional distress is a common risk in women with polycystic ovary syndrome: A systematic review and meta-analysis of 28 studies. *Human Reproduction Update, 18*(6), 638–651. https://doi.org/10.1093/humupd/dms029

Viloria, H. (2017). *Born both: An intersex life.* Hachette Books.

Viloria, H., & Nieto, M. (2020). *The spectrum of sex: The science of male, female, and intersex.* Jessica Kingsley Publishers.

Vujovic, S., Popovic, S., Sbutega-Milosevic, G., Djordjevic, M., & Gooren, L. (2009). Transsexualism in Serbia: A twenty-year follow-up study. *Journal of Sexual Medicine, 6*(4), 1018–1023. https://doi.org/10.1111/j.1743-6109.2008.00799.x

Ware, J. E., Jr., & Sherbourne, C. D. (1992). The MOS 36-item Short-Form Health Survey (SF-36). I. Conceptual framework and item selection. *Medical Care, 30*(6), 473–483. https://doi.org/10.1097/00005650-199206000-00002

Washington, R. (2008). The effect of polycystic ovary syndrome on the quality of life of pre-menopausal women. *Journal of the National Society of Allied Health, 5*(6), 8–22.

Webb, L., & Quennerstedt, M. (2010). Risky bodies: Health surveillance and teachers' embodiment of health. *International Journal of Qualitative Studies in Education: QSE, 23*(7), 785–802. https://doi.org/10.1080/09518398.2010.529471

Weeden, J., & Sabini, J. (2005). Physical attractiveness and health in Western societies: A review. *Psychological Bulletin, 131*(5), 635–653. https://doi.org/10.1037/0033-2909.131.5.635

Weir, C. B., & Jan, A. (2021). *BMI classification percentile and cut off points.* StatPearls Publishing.

Weiss, T. R., & Bulmer, S. M. (2011). Young women's experiences living with polycystic ovary syndrome. *JOGNN, 40*(6), 709–718. https://doi.org/10.1111/j.1552-6909.2011.01299.x

White-Davis, T., Edgoose, J., Brown Speights, J. S., Fraser, K., Ring, J. M., Guh, J., & Saba, G. W. (2018). Addressing racism in medical education: An interactive training module. *Family Medicine, 50*(5), 364–368. https://doi.org/10.22454/FamMed.2018.875510

Whiteford, L. M., & Gonzalez, L. (1995). Stigma: The hidden burden of infertility. *Social Science & Medicine, 40*(1), 27–36. https://doi.org/10.1016/0277-9536(94)00124-C

Wicks, S., Berger, Z., & Camic, P. M. (2019). It's how I am . . . it's what I am . . . it's a part of who I am: A narrative exploration of the impact of adolescent-onset chronic illness on identity formation in young people. *Clinical Child Psychology and Psychiatry, 24*(1), 40–52. https://doi.org/10.1177/1359104518818868

Wiederman, M. W. (2001). "Don't look now": The role of self-focus in sexual dysfunction. *The Family Journal, 9*(2), 210–214. https://doi.org/10.1177/1066480701092020

Wilkinson, S. (1988). The role of reflexivity in feminist psychology. *Women's Studies International Forum, 11*(5), 493–502. https://doi.org/10.1016/0277-5395(88)90024-6

Williams, S., Sheffield, D., & Knibb, R. C. (2015). "Everything's from the inside out with PCOS": Exploring women's experiences of living with polycystic ovary syndrome and co-morbidities through Skype™ interviews. *Health Psychology Open, 2*(2), 2055102915603051. https://doi.org/10.1177/2055102915603051

Williams, S., Sheffield, D., & Knibb, R. C. (2018). The polycystic ovary syndrome quality of life scale (PCOSQOL): Development and preliminary validation. *Health Psychology Open, 5*(2), 2055102918788195. https://doi.org/10.1177/2055102918788195

Williams, S. L., Fekete, E. M., & Skinta, M. D. (2021). Self-compassion in PLWH: Less internalized shame and negative psychosocial outcomes. *Behavioral Medicine, 47*(1), 60–68. https://doi.org/10.1080/08964289.2019.1659749

Williams, S. L., & Fredrick, E. G. (2015). One size may not fit all: The need for a more inclusive and intersectional psychology science on stigma. *Sex Roles, 73*(9–10), 384–390. https://doi.org/10.1007/s11199-015-0491-z

Williams, S. L., LaDuke, S. L., Klik, K., & Hutsell, D. W. (2016). A paradox of support seeking and support response among gays and lesbians. *Personal Relationships, 23*(2), 296–310. https://doi.org/10.1111/pere.12127

Winfrey, O., & Perry, B. D. (2021). *What happened to you?: Conversations on trauma, resilience, and healing.* Flatiron Books.

Wingo, E., Ingraham, N., & Roberts, S. C. M. (2018). Reproductive health care priorities and barriers to effective care for LGBTQ people assigned female at birth: A qualitative study. *Women's Health Issues, 28*(4), 350–357. https://doi.org/10.1016/j.whi.2018.03.002

Woertman, L., & van den Brink, F. (2012). Body image and female sexual functioning and behavior: A review. *Journal of Sex Research, 49*(2–3), 184–211. https://doi.org/10.1080/00224499.2012.658586

Wolf, W. M., Wattick, R. A., Kinkade, O. N., & Olfert, M. D. (2018). Geographical prevalence of polycystic ovary syndrome as determined by region and race/ethnicity. *International Journal of Environmental Research and Public Health, 15*(11), 2589–2602. https://doi.org/10.3390/ijerph15112589

Woods, N. F., & Kenney, N. J. (2019). Menstrual-cycle-related disorders: Polycystic ovary syndrome, dysmenorrhea and menstrual migraine. In J. M. Ussher, J. C. Chrisler, & J. Perz (Eds.), *Routledge international handbook of women's sexual and reproductive health* (pp. 101–126). Routledge. https://doi.org/10.4324/9781351035620-8

Woodward, A., Klonizakis, M., & Broom, D. (2020). Exercise and polycystic ovary syndrome. *Advances in Experimental Medicine and Biology, 1228*, 123–136. https://doi.org/10.1007/978-981-15-1792-1_8

World Health Organization. (1998). *WHOQOL user manual.*

World Health Organization. (n.d.). *WHO/Europe brief: Transgender health in the context of* ICD-11. https://www.who.int/standards/classifications/frequently-asked-questions/gender-incongruence-and-transgender-health-in-the-icd

Wright, P. J., Dawson, R. M., & Corbett, C. F. (2020). Social construction of biopsychosocial and medical experiences of women with polycystic ovary syndrome. *Journal of Advanced Nursing, 76*(7), 1728–1736. https://doi.org/10.1111/jan.14371

Wu, Y. K., & Berry, D. C. (2018). Impact of weight stigma on physiological and psychological health outcomes for overweight and obese adults: A systematic review. *Journal of Advanced Nursing, 74*(5), 1030–1042. https://doi.org/10.1111/jan.13511

Yildiz, B. O., Bolour, S., Woods, K., Moore, A., & Azziz, R. (2010). Visually scoring hirsutism. *Human Reproduction Update, 16*(1), 51–64. https://doi.org/10.1093/humupd/dmp024

Zhao, S., Wang, J., Xie, Q., Luo, L., Zhu, Z., Liu, Y., Luo, J., & Zhao, Z. (2019). Is polycystic ovary syndrome associated with risk of female sexual dysfunction? A systematic review and meta-analysis. *Reproductive Biomedicine Online, 38*(6), 979–989. https://doi.org/10.1016/j.rbmo.2018.11.030

Zinsser, W. (2013). *On writing well: The classic guide to writing nonfiction.* Collins.

Zueff, L. N., Lara, L. A., Vieira, C. S., Martins, W. P., & Ferriani, R. A. (2015). Body composition characteristics predict sexual functioning in obese women with or without PCOS. *Journal of Sex & Marital Therapy, 41*(3), 227–237. https://doi.org/10.1080/0092623X.2013.864369

Index

About the Author

Stacey L. Williams, PhD, is a social-health psychologist and professor in the Department of Psychology at East Tennessee State University (ETSU). She directs the Social Issues and Relations Laboratory, in which she and her students study stigma and health. She has published dozens of articles in this area, and her research has been funded by the National Institutes of Health. She teaches courses in topics related to diversity, gender and sexuality, and research methods and statistics. Currently, Dr. Williams serves as the chair of the campus institutional review board. Recent accomplishments include membership in the Leadership Institute for Women in Psychology and awards for both her research and equity and inclusion work: the ETSU College of Arts and Sciences Faculty Research Award, the Hayward Outstanding Psychology Faculty Award, the Notable Woman Award, and the Patricia E. Robertson Diversity Leadership Award. Before her professorship, she earned her PhD in psychology at Kent State University and completed a postdoctoral research fellowship in social environment and health at the Institute for Social Research, University of Michigan.